'I wish there had been such a clea[obscured]
this when I received my diagnosi[obscured]
rebuild myself after treatment had finished. Life changes after cancer, and with Rosamund's amazing recommendations, we really can thrive.'

Sarah Newman, cancer fitness specialist

'Rosamund is dedicated to improving the lives and experiences of people with breast cancer and this book is a tremendous collection of helpful tips for those embarking on, going through or coming out the other side of treatment. I look forward to sharing it with my patients.'

Kat Tunnicliffe, oncological physiotherapist

'Having a breast cancer diagnosis can be a lonely and overwhelming experience, and there is an overload of information right from the start. Rosamund's book is not only the manual I wish I'd had, but also warm, funny and kind. It's like having a big sister who has been through the same thing, right by your side. Informative and calming, *Reconstruction* should be prescribed at the moment of that frightening diagnosis. Thank you, from the bottom of my heart.'

Sarah Cawood, broadcaster

'Rosamund writes with a style that makes you feel you're having a chat with a good friend – a warm, clever and vivacious friend. In *Reconstruction,* Rosamund has brilliantly summarised a wealth of information into bitesize, digestible pieces, and called attention to important subjects that are often overlooked within cancer care, such as the benefits of movement.'

Emily Jenkins, founder of Move Dance Feel

'Rosamund has left no stone unturned in this comprehensive, informative and practical guide for those affected by breast cancer. I like the fact that there is clear signposting to many valuable resources for every stage of the breast cancer experience. I wish I had this book at my bedside when I was diagnosed 26 years ago.'

Marcia Mercier, yoga for breast cancer teacher

'Brilliant! Rosamund Dean has just made it easier to navigate the complexities of living through and beyond a breast cancer diagnosis. This book leads the reader through treatment options and, importantly, how to stay healthy once treatment is over.'

Emma Holly, scar therapist

'I wish a book like this had been given to me when diagnosed. It would have been the companion I absolutely needed to navigate the craziness of a breast cancer diagnosis and will support so many as they face their own frightening diagnosis.'

Carly Moosah, breast cancer campaigner

'I am beyond delighted that Rosamund has decided to write about the significant impact of menopause alongside all the other important matters in her fabulous new book *Reconstruction*. True healing and recovery after cancer cannot take place without addressing some of the symptoms that come with menopause. This book is a true resource powerhouse and one you would want on your bedside table for sure!'

Dani Binnington, host of
The Menopause and Cancer Podcast

re con struction

How to rebuild your body, mind and life after a **breast cancer** diagnosis

ROSAMUND DEAN

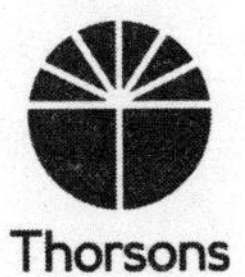

This book contains advice and information relating to health care. It should be used to supplement rather than replace the advice of your doctor or another trained health professional. If you know or suspect you have a health problem, it is recommended that you seek your doctor's advice before embarking on any medical programme or treatment. All efforts have been made to assure the accuracy of the information contained in this book as of the date of publication. This publisher and the author disclaim liability for any medical outcomes that may occur as a result of applying the methods suggested in this book.

Thorsons
An imprint of HarperCollins*Publishers*
1 London Bridge Street
London SE1 9GF

www.harpercollins.co.uk

HarperCollins*Publishers*
Macken House, 39/40 Mayor Street Upper
Dublin 1, D01 C9W8, Ireland

First published by Thorsons 2023

10 9 8 7 6 5 4 3 2 1

Illustrations: p.256, 259 Nicolas Primola/Shutterstock.com; p.257 Katule/Shutterstock.com; p.258 (top) solar22/Shutterstock.com; p.258 (bottom) Lio Putra/Shutterstock.com

A catalogue record of this book is available from the British Library

ISBN 978-0-00-858520-4

Printed and bound in the UK using 100% renewable electricity at CPI Group (UK) Ltd

This book is produced from independently certified FSC™ paper to ensure responsible forest management.

For more information visit: www.harpercollins.co.uk/green

For Jonathan

Contents

Introduction

My right breast was not the only thing that cancer took from me. I have also had to reconstruct my entire lifestyle, my mindset and my identity.

Before breast cancer, I was one of those people that never got ill, never went to the doctor and didn't even like to take a painkiller for a headache if I could help it. I was so certain of my general good health that when I found a lump on my right breast just before Christmas 2020, I felt completely sure that it must be a cyst or some hormonal thing related to having just turned 40.

My subsequent diagnosis in January 2021 was a shock. But, looking at the statistics, perhaps it shouldn't have been. In 2020, breast cancer had the dubious honour of displacing lung cancer to become the most diagnosed cancer worldwide. Here in the UK, it's also the most common cancer overall, with one in seven women diagnosed in their lifetime. According to statistics from Cancer Research UK, there are around 57,000 new breast cancer cases every year; more than 150 a day, so effectively one every 10 minutes. And it's not merely the realm of the over-50s any more. Since the early 1990s, breast cancer rates in 25–49-year-old women have increased by 17 per cent. It is now the leading cause of death for women aged 35–49 in the UK. Let's say that again; it is now the leading cause of death for women aged 35–49.

When I wrote about my experience of breast cancer treatment in a column for the *Sunday Times Style* magazine I was blown away by the response. The column, which was co-written with my husband, Jonathan, ran for a year and covered everything from getting through chemotherapy, mastectomy surgery and radiotherapy, to how I coped with the psychological trauma of losing my hair and the anxiety about my risk of recurrence. It also dug into the impact on my family, which is why it was so interesting to write alongside Jonathan. I received hundreds of emails and direct messages from readers saying that the column had articulated how they felt, and helped them to feel less alone. I found this heartbreaking because a breast cancer diagnosis and the treatment that follows is extremely tough, and no one should ever have to cope with that alone. Isolation was even more prevalent during the Covid pandemic, for obvious reasons.

I have since learned that there are many resources available, although they are not always easy to find, which is one of the reasons that I wanted to write this book.

The good news is that while diagnosis rates are on the rise, breast cancer survival rates are improving, and have doubled in the last 40 years. So I know that there are hundreds of thousands of us out there, needing warm, relatable advice for getting through treatment and rebuilding ourselves afterwards. This is a pragmatic-but-positive book for people going through breast cancer, and their families and friends. It's a sensible guide, but I've tried to make it optimistic and hopeful, sharing positive advice for breast cancer patients and their supporters, while looking forward to a healthy long life after cancer. If you like, this is the cancer equivalent of one of those pregnancy books, with clear advice on what to expect at every stage of treatment and what questions to ask your doctors, right down to what to pack in your hospital bag. Think of it as a guide to what to expect when you're expecting the worst.

After writing the column, many readers contacted me asking for advice about their own situation, and they still do. I'm not a doctor, but, having been through the breast cancer mill, I now know the process from the inside out. And, as a journalist, I'm used to interviewing experts and translating sometimes-impenetrable medical advice, statistics and information in a way that is clear and useful for a wider audience.

As well as being an emotional support, you'll find practical advice here for all the stages of treatment, and further ways in which you can reduce your risk of recurrence. An estimated quarter of all breast cancer cases in the UK are preventable and, while no one can claim to prevent cancer completely (there are just too many varied causes, many of which are not yet fully understood), there are certainly steps that you can take to reduce your risk.

I want you to be able to flick quickly to the part of this book that you most need right now, so it's broken down into four parts. Dip in and out as required. The idea is that, if you're struggling with overwhelm, fatigue and brain fog caused by cancer treatment and its side effects, you can go straight to what you need at that moment and ignore everything else.

Part I: Diagnosis

An introduction to the different types of breast cancer and the people you will meet as part of your medical team. It also covers advice about coming to terms with your diagnosis psychologically, and what additional tools and resources are available to support you through treatment.

Part II: Treatment

The most practical chapter, taking each element of treatment in turn, and explaining what you need to know. Everyone's experience is different, so whether you need chemotherapy, surgery, radiotherapy, hormonal therapy, targeted treatments or all of the above, you can turn to the page most relevant for you.

Part III: The end of treatment and the myth of the all-clear

Here I address post-treatment issues like menopausal symptoms and fear of recurrence, as well as a positive report on the future of cancer treatment. Then, there's a guide to designing your new identity and stepping into your post-cancer life feeling renewed rather than decimated. It might not feel like it yet, but this *is* possible. *If you are newly diagnosed, you might not want to read this section until you're closer to it, but it's here when you're ready.*

Part IV: Future-proofing your body

Once you've been through cancer treatment, I'm fairly certain you'll be keen to do anything and everything to avoid ever having to do it again. There are plenty of steps you can take to reduce your risk of recurrence, and new treatment breakthroughs are happening all the time. This is your guide.

Throughout the book, I often refer to women because men account for less than 1 per cent of breast cancer cases. But this can be a particularly difficult diagnosis for men, who may feel a sense of shame about having what is considered a 'female' type of cancer. If you are a man with breast cancer, the sections on hormonal issues and the menopause will not be so relevant, but hopefully you can still get a lot out of this book. In fact, if you don't have breast cancer but have a family history or a loved one going through it, you'll find much that is helpful here too.

This book is for anyone whose life has been touched by breast cancer, and it's the book I wish I'd had by my bedside when I was diagnosed. I hope that it helps you.

PART I:
DIAGNOSIS

My Story

In December 2020, cancer was the last thing on my mind. I had a busy, fun job as deputy editor of *Grazia* magazine. My husband Jonathan and I have two kids, Ezra and Eden, who were then six and three, and we were busy with pre-Christmas deadlines and the usual festive stress that time of year can bring. So when I felt a lump on my right breast one day, I almost didn't go to the doctor.

Since I am now such an advocate of regular breast-checking, I'm a bit embarrassed to admit that I did not routinely check my own breasts, and found the lump as a pure fluke while moisturising after a shower. According to Google, lumpy breasts are common and only one in ten lumps turns out to be cancer. It was Jonathan who nudged me to make sure I was going to call the surgery. And, when the appointment time came, I was having second thoughts. 'I can't even really feel it now,' I muttered. 'If I go, I'll be wasting the NHS's time during a pandemic.' (Oh yes, you might remember, there was a pandemic on at that time.)

'Well, you've made the appointment now,' replied Jonathan, 'so you're wasting their time if you *don't* go.'

The doctor could certainly feel the lump. Two days before Christmas, I was sitting in an East London breast clinic, replying to work emails and texting reassurances to Jonathan, in between being led into various rooms. First for a mammogram, then an ultrasound, and eventually a biopsy. Even then, I wasn't particularly concerned. Google assured me that four out of five breast biopsies come back benign. People with cancer are tired and ill-looking, I reasoned to myself. I was a healthy 40-year-old with neither the time nor the inclination to have cancer, thanks. If anything, I was just a bit frustrated at how long all this was taking.

After all the tests, the nurse said I had to see the doctor one last time before leaving, and I took a seat in his office as he nodded hello. The nurse also came into the room and, looking back, that should have been a clue that things were about to get more serious than I'd anticipated. This being the pandemic, we were all wearing blue surgical masks, so I couldn't see much of the doctor's face. He started explaining that biopsy results normally take a week but, because of Christmas and New Year, it would be two weeks.

'Of course, fine,' I nodded.

'So,' he continued, 'in January we will discuss whether to go straight to surgery or if you need to have chemotherapy first.'

Wait. What? I laughed awkwardly, but he didn't seem to be joking.

'But ... that's if it's cancer,' I said slowly. 'Which it might not be.'

'We can tell from the ultrasound that it's very likely to be cancer,' he said.

'How likely?'

'Ninety-five per cent.'

The worst news of my life, delivered in a brutally casual way. Hot tears formed and were absorbed into my face covering. The nurse, perhaps feeling that the doctor's manner had been a bit brusque, ushered me into another room. She explained that breast lumps are given a cancer-likelihood score out of five, known as BI-RADS (for breast imaging and reporting data system). Mine was a five, meaning the growth was highly likely to be malignant.

'I have seen people with a score of five get a benign biopsy result,' she said. 'It does happen.'

'Oh right, okay.' I sniffed.

'Well, a very small number,' she back-pedalled, realising she'd given me foundation-less hope. 'In most cases, it is cancer.'

I called Jonathan as soon as I left the hospital but, perhaps due to shock, I only told him that I'd had a biopsy and would get the results in two weeks. I didn't mention what the doctor had said until I got home. By that point, I had pulled myself together, and we both agreed not to spiral into panic, at least until we knew for sure. It's an odd feeling, being told a life-changing diagnosis is probably on the horizon but not yet confirmed.

The next two weeks passed in a daze of shell-shocked calm. Jonathan and I were torn between trying to come to terms with a cancer diagnosis, and hoping that I'd be in the 5 per cent of biopsies that turn out to be fine.

We decided not to tell anyone before the biopsy result, which was actually easy since Covid restrictions meant we weren't allowed to see anyone anyway. We didn't want to worry our families, particularly our children, until we really had to. So we opened Christmas presents, made a nut roast and cheerily FaceTimed my mum, who lives in Scotland and was shielding with a chronic chest condition. When we became tearful, we blamed whichever Pixar movie we had just watched with the kids.

On 6 January, I was back in the breast clinic to receive the results. It was pretty clear that bad news was coming when, on the phone, they said I could bring someone with me. Thanks to Covid restrictions, this was one of only two or three times when I was allowed to have Jonathan in the room with me, over the following months of tests, appointments, chemotherapy and surgery. We are both pretty calm in a crisis, or maybe we were in shock, but we nodded politely as it was explained that, yes, it is cancer. The surgeon (thankfully, a different doctor to the short-shrift one from before Christmas) said the cancer was 'triple negative'. Having never heard of that before, I looked at him blankly before asking: 'Is that a good thing or a bad thing?'

He shrugged. 'It's not really good or bad, it's just a type of breast cancer.' There were two separate tumours in the breast (this is known as multifocal cancer), and the ultrasound had suggested lymph node involvement, which was quickly confirmed with another biopsy, so I would need five months of chemotherapy before I could have surgery. We were so dazed that we didn't ask many questions, but the one I do remember asking is: 'Can I assure my kids that I'm not going to die?' I cried with relief when the answer was 'Yes'. Looking back, this was before they had done the MRI, CT and bone scans to check that there was no cancer elsewhere in my body, so they can't have known that for sure, but I still feel grateful they said it. We were handed leaflets and told to expect appointment dates for all of those scans and the first of many oncological appointments. I wasn't to see a surgeon again until much closer to my surgery date, in the summer.

The next couple of hours were spent walking around a freezing park, calling my family and closest friends to let them know. I started each conversation with a jaunty: 'So I've got some news that *sounds* bad, but it's going to be *fine*.' My mum lives alone and had lost her sister to ovarian cancer only a few months earlier, so I arranged for a local friend to pop by for a doorstep chat with her immediately after I broke the news. Being 400 miles away, it was hard that I couldn't hug her. But, because of the restrictions, I wasn't even allowed to hug my friend who lives around the corner. It's one of many reasons why I felt so grateful to have Jonathan and the kids during the following year. I can't imagine what it must have been like for people who live alone, dealing with a cancer diagnosis during the pandemic.

I understand that many people make the decision to keep their diagnosis quiet, only telling friends and family on a need-to-know basis, and I can certainly see the appeal of not having people constantly asking how you are, or feeling as though you're the morbidly fascinating topic of conversation among colleagues, acquaintances and extended family. For me, keeping it quiet would have felt stressful, as though I was carrying a secret. As a journalist, I was already active on social media, sharing career and family highs and lows on Instagram, so it made sense to me to share the news on there – but only after I had talked to close friends and family directly. I liked the sense of community on Instagram, and welcomed support and advice on the platform. As with many stages in the breast cancer journey, this will be a case of working out what's best for you.

Over the previous two weeks of probably-cancer, I had read a lot online about the best way to talk to young children about this kind of diagnosis, and decided to be totally honest. If we had tried to hide it they'd hear us talking and pick up on it anyway. Particularly since the government had just announced the third national lockdown, thanks to a new, more-transmissible Covid variant, so the four of us were together all day every day.

At just six, Ezra was old enough to have known people die of cancer, so I wanted to be clear with both of our kids that my diagnosis would be nothing like my aunt's experience. My cancer is treatable, and it will get better, I told them. I think it was the right approach. They took the news in that matter-of-fact way that children deal with everything, and we kept an open dialogue so that they could ask any questions, no matter how silly, at any point. To be honest, they didn't ask many, and I was glad that they were capable of accepting all manner of events as perfectly normal. I, on the other hand, was starting to realise my life was going to change quite dramatically over the next year.

I had left my job to go freelance in the week of my diagnosis, but this was actually coincidental rather than a direct result of having cancer. I had handed in my notice three months previously because, like a massive pandemic cliché, I'd reassessed my values in lockdown and decided that I wanted to work more flexibly to be around for the kids. There followed a flurry of financial panic. Had I stayed in a staff job, I would have been entitled to paid sick leave. As a freelancer, I was now in a situation where, if I didn't work then I didn't get paid.

Happily, I was asked to write the column for the *Sunday Times Style* magazine, and a few other bits and bobs that I could do on the days I felt up to it. It was certainly a pay-cut, but it's not as if I was having nights out or eating lavish meals at this point. I tried to see that year as a bit like a really depressing maternity leave – I wasn't earning much, but I also wasn't spending much, and I was lucky enough to have a partner who would still make sure the mortgage got paid. I had snapped into practical, businesslike mode and, to an outsider, would have looked like I was coping brilliantly. But a couple of weeks later, after blood work, a CT scan and an MRI, I felt like a lab rat, being endlessly jabbed with needles. And I'm one of those people with difficult-to-find veins, so it always took several tries. I veered wildly between apologising profusely to nurses for my terrible veins and getting quite short tempered when they couldn't get the cannula in.

In fact, my moods were suddenly all over the place. I got irrationally angry about details such as not being allowed to hug the kids after being injected with a radioactive tracer for the bone scan. I started snapping at Jonathan, and crying after each test, particularly when my (by now quite mangled) veins had taken another battering. I've always thought of myself as a sensible, rational – but generally positive – person. If anyone had tried to offer me psychological support at this point, I would have brushed them away with a smiley 'I'm fine'. But I do wish someone had started talking to me about the psychological impact of a cancer diagnosis, or even just explained to me what to expect at an MRI scan (naively, I didn't even know it involved a cannula).

While I'm immensely grateful to the NHS for saving my life, I also started to feel frustrated at the lack of information and options given to cancer patients. The doctor's vague reply to my question about triple negative breast cancer, and lack of forthcomingness in explaining what it is, meant that – obviously – I went home and googled it. I even optimistically thought, in medical situations, the word 'negative' is often a good thing, right?

What I actually learned (through Google alone) was that the prognosis for triple negative is worse than for other types of breast cancer, with a higher risk of recurrence. I felt sick as I read the stories of women who'd been diagnosed with triple negative breast cancer, all of which seemed to end badly. I could not understand why the doctor hadn't explained all this to me at the time. Did he think I wouldn't google it? As I learned more about triple negative breast cancer (or TNBC), I realised that treatments have improved a lot in recent years, and are getting better all the time. One oncologist even told me that my diagnosis would have been 'a death sentence' had it happened just 10 years earlier. No wonder I had stumbled across so many scary stats online. All that fear could have been avoided if the doctor had just taken five minutes to explain my own situation fully as an individual, unique patient.

A week after my diagnosis, I had a call from the surgeon to explain that further analysis of the biopsy showed my cancer was grade three, the fastest-growing type. This meant that, regardless of how well chemotherapy worked, they would have to do a mastectomy, so remove my entire breast, rather than perform breast-conserving surgery such as a lumpectomy. I remember hanging up from the call and thinking, right, so I've got the most aggressive grade of the most aggressive type of breast cancer? This was turning out to be much scarier than I'd imagined back when a friend assured me 'loads of celebrities get breast cancer, and it's like a thing for a year, and then they're fine!' I was also terrified about losing my breast, because nobody had told me about reconstruction options. If you'd have said the words 'DIEP flap' to me then, I would have been very confused. Now, having emerged from the other side of successful treatment for primary breast cancer, I want to demystify the whole process for other people.

Your support handbook

It was not only clear medical facts that I found hard to come by. Aside from a very welcome Macmillan Cancer Support call, I was told very little about what support services are available to cancer patients. I was a month into chemo before a nurse casually mentioned that I might want to wait for my blood test results in the hospital's Maggie's centre, rather than in the grim chemo waiting room. I remember walking into the beautifully light and airy building, with cosy sofas and bowls of biscuits on the blonde-wood tables. Within seconds, I'd been offered a cup of tea and given information about the courses they run. I couldn't help thinking: Why didn't anyone tell me about this place before? There are 26 Maggie's centres in the UK, all conveniently located on hospital grounds, often with beautiful gardens or terraces and all with warm, friendly, informed staff. If there's one near you, make sure you're using it.

And do ask your breast care nurse about what additional support there is available at your hospital, as cancer centres generally have access to psychologists and sometimes even complementary therapies such as reiki or reflexology. The options vary around the country but, in many places, it's a case of: if you don't ask, then you don't get.

I was also disappointed with the lack of advice from my medical team about any lifestyle steps you can take, and complementary therapies on offer, to help ease the brutal side effects of chemo, and even to reduce your risk of recurrence. The medical approach was very much focused on curing or managing the disease, rather than prevention and living cancer-free long-term. Yes, lots of this information exists online, but it's hard to know what's reputable. It took a lot of asking around, and trial and error, before I found what worked for me. I wanted that advice to come from my medical team because, as I mentioned, I'm a rational person. I need data and stats to prove to me that something works and, at the time, I thought complementary therapies were generally a money-making scam.

If you'd have asked me about the best cancer treatments at any point before my own diagnosis, I would have said the medical treatment prescribed by your doctor. It wouldn't even have crossed my mind to consider that some complementary therapies can have powerful effects. I was extremely cynical and, don't get me wrong, there are certainly unscrupulous people out there peddling expensive snake oil to terrified cancer patients. But now I've learned that many of these therapies can actually have enormous benefits, working alongside conventional medical treatment, and I wish I'd known about them sooner. If you're as cynical as I was, then do try and keep an open mind when we come to those.

Take something as simple as exercise, for example. Everyone knows it's good for you, but it's often talked about in terms of weight loss or *looking* fit. It wasn't until very late in my treatment that I learned how important it is for recovery and general health improvement outcomes. Exercise can ease side effects during chemotherapy, and even reduce your risk of recurrence by up to an astounding 55 per cent. But not one doctor mentioned it to me. I learned about these benefits through social media – after establishing which accounts were sharing evidence-based information. However, without more specific advice, I threw myself into yoga a few months after surgery and actually brought on lymphoedema (*see page 109*) in my right arm with too many planks and downward dogs.

Nobody had told me that I shouldn't put my body weight on my wrists so soon after lymph node removal.

With my journalistic background, I was probably an incredibly annoying patient, asking more questions than I imagine doctors are used to. The good news is that I can share what I've learned. This can be your handbook, to make your journey through breast cancer treatment and beyond easier and clearer. I want to simplify everything about the process, laying out all the information I wish I'd had from the beginning, in the order that you need it.

Your Medical Team

It's important to understand the different roles of people that you will meet along the way, and to get the most out of your short face-to-face (or telephone) sessions with these busy experts. Initially, I thought of everyone I met as a 'doctor' and would constantly be asking the wrong person the wrong question.

You might assume that there is some kind of a 'project manager' who has an overview of your full treatment plan, and who will guide you through the various aspects of your care. Sadly, this is not the case, which is why it's important that you understand the person you're speaking to has expertise in their own field, but often can't advise on anything outside their remit. I want to make your life easier by helping you ask the right questions of the right people.

From the moment that you are diagnosed with breast cancer, there is a whole team of people working to help you. There's your surgeon, your medical and clinical oncologists and, in the background, there are people like radiologists interpreting scans and pathologists who analyse the blood tests. Some of those people you'll meet as you need them, some you'll never meet at all, but they're a key part of your treatment pathway. Most cancer units have a multidisciplinary team (MDT) meeting every week, so everyone in your wider medical team should be up-to-date on your progress. The following few sections explain each role clearly, so you know who you'll be meeting, and what to expect from them.

Your breast surgeon

In most cases, surgery is the single most important thing you can do to get rid of your cancer. Other treatments, which we'll come to, can be used to shrink your tumour before surgery. This is known as neoadjuvant therapy. And further treatments can be used to reduce your risk of recurrence by blitzing any stray cancer cells that may remain in your body after surgery. This is known as adjuvant therapy. But it all revolves around the surgery that will literally cut the cancer out of your body.

Your surgeon will be the first person you meet from your medical team. It will be your surgeon who breaks the news that the symptom you've been worried about is, in fact, cancer. For this appointment, when your diagnosis is explained to you for the first time, they may suggest in advance that you bring someone with you. This is a good idea for all of those early surgical and oncological appointments. If you can, always take someone along because, as soon as you hear the words 'you have cancer', your brain fails to take in anything else. You need another pair of ears at most of those initial planning appointments, and another person to ask questions that you might not think of in the moment as your brain scrambles to keep up. And you can always record the meeting on your phone to listen to later, if you need to.

Whether you have surgery before or after chemotherapy, or only surgery without the need for chemo, will depend on several factors. These include the type of breast cancer (more on which shortly) and the stage and grade of the tumour.

STAGES

Most people know that stage four means the cancer has spread (or metastasised) from the breast into another part of the body. Once this has happened, there is no cure, and treatment is designed to manage the cancer for the rest of your life. This is known as secondary, or metastatic, breast cancer, and people can live with it for years. (For more information on this, turn to the chapter on secondary breast cancer, *page 214*.)

The majority of breast cancers are diagnosed between stages one to three, known as primary breast cancer, and can be treated with curative intent.

Here's how the stages are defined:

Stage one usually means that the cancer is small and contained within the breast.

Stage two usually means that the tumour is slightly larger but hasn't started to spread into the surrounding tissues. Sometimes stage two means that cancer cells have spread into the lymph nodes under your arm (known as axillary lymph nodes).

Stage three means the cancer is larger again. It may have started to spread into surrounding tissue, and there are cancer cells in the axillary lymph nodes.

Here in the UK, you might also hear people talking about T1 and T2 tumours. This is simply another way of describing the stage of the cancer using the TNM system, which stands for tumour, node and metastasis.

- T1 means that the tumour is two centimetres across or less.
- T2 means that the tumour is more than two centimetres but no more than five centimetres.
- T3 means the tumour, or tumours, are bigger than five centimetres across.
- T4 means the tumour has spread to another part of the body, or is inflammatory.

For example, my breast cancer was stage three because there were two separate tumours in the same breast (this is known as multifocal); one nearly four centimetres, and the other slightly smaller, so a total mass of around seven centimetres. There were also cancer cells identified in two of my right axillary lymph nodes. Had I only had one tumour, then it might have been considered stage two, even with lymph node involvement.

Grading is from one to three, with three being the fastest-growing. If your tumour is grade three, as mine was, don't panic, that's not necessarily a bad thing. More aggressive tumours can often react better to treatment than slower-growing ones.

TYPES OF BREAST CANCER

This is where it gets complicated. I have seen people's eyes glaze over when they've asked me what my diagnosis of 'triple negative' means and I've launched into a description. You can't really describe triple negative breast cancer without first explaining other types of breast cancer, as it is defined by not having those features. The main types of breast cancer that you will hear about are categorised by the proteins and hormone receptors that are present (or not) in the tumour. Here's a rundown of them:

- **Hormone receptor positive** cancers include **ER+**, where the cancer cells contain oestrogen receptors, and **PR+**, where the cells contain progesterone receptors (although PR+ tumours are usually also ER+). These account for around 75 per cent of cases. As well as surgery, radiotherapy and/or chemotherapy where necessary, they can be treated with hormone treatments, also known as endocrine therapy. These include tamoxifen, letrozole and Zoladex.
- **HER2** breast cancer means that the cells have a high level of human epidermal growth factor receptor 2. This accounts for around 10–15 per cent of cases and can be treated with targeted drugs like Herceptin and Perjeta, often given in combination as an injection called Phesgo.

- **Triple negative breast cancer** (or TNBC) means that none of the three factors above apply, so the cancer is oestrogen and progesterone receptor negative and HER2 negative. This also accounts for around 10–15 per cent of cases, and is most common in young (by which I mean premenopausal) women. People with TNBC are more likely to have an inherited gene mutation and will usually be offered a blood test to check for mutations in the genes BRCA1 and BRCA2. If you have genetic testing, there are other less common mutations such as TP53, PALB2, ATM and CHEK2, so it's good to be tested for as many as you can. Traditionally, there have been fewer targeted treatments available for TNBC than there have been for other types of breast cancer, although, in 2022, an immunotherapy drug called pembrolizumab was approved for use within the NHS, improving outcomes for patients with primary TNBC.
- Within these categories, there are many more factors to consider. For example, HER2-low cancers can be hormone receptor positive *or* triple negative, and different targeted treatments (such as the relatively new drug Enhertu) can work in that instance. And, yes, if the tumour is ER+, PR+ and HER2+, it's described as triple positive – which means you could get the triple whammy of chemo, Phesgo and hormonal treatments. That sounds grim, but it's really giving you the very best chance of zapping your cancer for good.

- You may also hear people talk about **lobular** or **ductal** breast cancer, which simply describes where the cancer originated. Lobular breast cancer is less common, and it starts in the cells that line the lobules (or glands where breastmilk is produced), rather than in the ducts, which are the little tubes that carry milk to the nipple. This is important to be aware of, if only because lobular breast cancer rarely presents as a lump. It's more likely to be a thickening or swelling of the skin, or a change in the nipple such as becoming inverted. Then there are rarer types, such as inflammatory breast cancer, where the cancer cells have blocked lymph ducts in the breast, so it may become red, swollen and hot to touch. Treatment for these cancers will still depend on the proteins and hormone receptors, as above.

I know that sounds confusing, and you absolutely do not need to know everything about every type of breast cancer. But it's good to be aware of the differences, so that you can get relevant-for-you information, otherwise it can be easy to get bogged down and overwhelmed. Focus on getting through your own treatment, and try not to compare your experience to other people's. There are so many different variables and factors at play and, while it's good to understand the different treatment options available and keep an open dialogue with your oncologist and surgeon, you should also trust in the process.

If you have private healthcare, you have a choice to make.

Some people with private health insurance decide to be treated on the NHS as, soon after the initial diagnosis, they may find things moving quickly and feel that switching to private care might actually slow the process down. Also, there is sometimes a financial incentive from health insurers if you access care on the NHS, which can be important if you're taking a long period off work. In my case, I didn't have private health insurance, and was gutted to learn that a new immunotherapy treatment was available privately for TNBC, which was not yet being used within the NHS. Since then, that drug (pembrolizumab) has been approved for NHS use. So, had I been diagnosed two years later, my treatment would have been pretty similar whether private or NHS. Everyone's situation is different, so it must be your decision.

DIAGNOSTIC SCANS

By the time you pick up this book, you will probably already have had a mammogram and an ultrasound before the biopsy to diagnose your breast cancer. After diagnosis, you will likely then have other scans, the purpose of which is to check that the cancer has not spread elsewhere in the body. Don't worry if you don't have all of these; different doctors prefer different types of scan. For example, throughout my entire diagnosis and treatment, I have never had a PET scan, which my oncologist said was not necessary if I'd had an MRI and CT. Ask your surgeon or oncologist about their decisions on the scans they have advised in your particular case. Here is a quick need-to-know rundown for each of them.

Mammogram: An X-ray for breasts, during which you are naked from the waist up. The mammographer will place your breast onto the machine, and it will be squeezed between two pieces of plastic to keep it still while the X-rays are taken.

Ultrasound: The sonographer will put ultrasound gel onto the skin, and then move the probe across it, while high-frequency sound waves produce an image of the inside of your breast. This can assess a larger area than the mammogram.

MRI: Magnetic resonance imaging takes pictures of your breast tissue using magnetic fields and radio waves. You will have a cannula in your arm or hand, through which a contrast dye is injected during the scan. The dye helps create clearer images that outline abnormalities more easily.

CT scan: Like an MRI, computerised tomography scans are useful after your diagnosis to look for any breast cancer deposits (or metastases) elsewhere in the body. Again, you will have a cannula inserted to administer a contrast dye that shows up body tissues more clearly.

PET scan: Positron emission tomography scans allow doctors to see metabolic processes in the body, and any disturbance of these processes by disease. A PET scan is often carried out alongside a CT scan, known as a PET/CT.

Your plastic surgeon

Depending on what kind of surgery you have, and if you want reconstruction after a mastectomy, you may also meet a plastic surgeon. Their specialism is making your body feel like yours again. NHS care has come on leaps and bounds in this area, and your team should be sensitive and aware of the psychological trauma of losing one or both breasts.

Most people will meet their breast surgeon and their plastic surgeon separately but, if you're lucky, you may get one of the handful of surgeons in the UK to be trained in both plastic surgery and breast surgical oncology.

Miss Georgette Oni (surgeons are bizarrely always 'Miss' or 'Mr' rather than 'Doctor') is one of them, specialising in oncoplastic breast surgery at the Nottingham Breast Institute. Initially training as a plastic surgeon specialising in reconstruction, she expanded her remit because she wanted to be involved in patient care from the beginning. 'I truly believe that if all the elements are there at your diagnosis, then you're more likely to have the best possible journey, during what is already a very difficult time,' she says. 'Where I work, we have three plastic surgeons that do breast oncology, but it's actually very rare to have that. Which is a shame because studies show that if your breast unit is attached to a plastic surgery unit, it opens up the choices that patients have, and it makes such a difference to their experience of reconstruction.'

My personal experience speaks to this, because I found that my breast surgeon told me one thing, then it would take a week to get an appointment with the plastic surgeon, who would tell me something different. Having the same person cover both areas, or even speaking to them together would have been brilliant.

'It's a big issue, plastics and breast surgeons not being in the same room,' Miss Oni says with a nod. 'In Nottingham, even if you don't have the plastic surgeon and the breast surgeon in one person, we actually do all of our reconstructive clinics together anyway. Unfortunately, there are many more breast units than there are plastic surgery units so, in some parts of the country, your plastic surgery unit might be 20 or 30 miles away from where you live.'

If this is the case for you, then don't feel as though you have to rush into any decision about surgery. Give yourself time to speak to your plastics team and think about your options, before making sure that you are completely happy. The plastics team is there to put you back together again, which is rather an important job. Should you want them to, of course. Some women prefer to have an aesthetic flat closure.

'If you don't want to have reconstruction, then you'll be flat and there will be scarring,' says Miss Oni. 'But, with the latest techniques, we try to make that scar sit as flat and as low as we can, because that helps with overall aesthetics, and also in terms of prosthesis fitting if you choose to do that.'

For this type of surgery, you're unlikely to need a plastic surgeon, as most breast surgeons will be conversant with the appropriate oncoplastic techniques to improve the aesthetic look of your flat closure.

All of this will be a conversation that you have with your surgical team. To illustrate how far we've come, my nan was diagnosed with breast cancer at a young age (in the 1950s) and she had no option of reconstruction. She described not fully understanding the surgery she was about to undergo and, believing that they were just removing the tumour, was shocked to wake up and learn they had removed her entire breast. There was no conversation at all about the psychological impact. She was given a beanbag to put in her bra, and sent home. Of course, she just got on with it, and my mum remembers the beanbag drying on the radiator when she was a child. However, after Nan's second diagnosis in the 1990s, when reconstruction was an option, she was much older and announced that she would rather go flat and wear a vest 'like a man'. It breaks my heart to think of her putting a beanbag in her bra, when she might have been so much happier with reconstruction, or even the option of a risk-reducing bilateral mastectomy (even back then, we had a family history of breast cancer).

These days, reconstruction takes many forms. 'In terms of total reconstruction, your options are either using a foreign body or using your own body,' explains Miss Oni. 'A foreign body is obviously an implant, and using your own body is called autologous reconstruction.'

The best-known type of autologous reconstruction is DIEP flap (*see also page 92*), where the new breast is moulded out of fat from another part of your body, usually the abdomen. Both options have pros and cons, although using your own tissue has been shown to result in greater satisfaction with the results long-term. However, the vast majority of people still have implants. Why? Well, for one thing, not everywhere has access to plastic surgeons able to perform DIEP flap reconstruction, so that might not even be a conversation for them. Also, you need to have enough abdominal tissue to create the new breast, so very slender women might not have it as an option. Nevertheless, you can also take tissue from other parts of the body, such as the thigh, bum, back or even the love handles, if there isn't enough elsewhere.

'Also, we find that a lot of our younger patients will choose implants, even though they have an autologous option,' reveals Miss Oni. 'It's often because they want a quicker recovery, which you get with implants because you're not taking bits from other parts of the body. Or they don't want to have the scar across their abdomen.'

Those are two excellent reasons, so why is long-term satisfaction greater with DIEP flap? 'The trouble with implant-based reconstruction is that your body knows it's a foreign body,' explains Miss Oni. 'So it creates a wall around it called a capsule. With time, that capsule can become tight and change the shape and feel of the breasts. It's called capsular contracture and, if you have radiotherapy, it can speed up that process. The other thing is that there can be issues with implants that mean coming back and forth for other operations over the course of your lifetime.'

The main thing for Miss Oni – and hopefully for your surgeon too – is that you are happy with the results. She tells me her aim is not only the patient's survival, but also their ability to live well after surgery. 'If every time they take their clothes off, they are confronted with a terrible-looking scar or a really poor reconstruction, it will have a very long-lasting effect on their psyche,' she says. 'We are always working on new techniques for making sure that the reconstruction or closure is as pleasant on the eye as possible, because it will be looked at on a daily basis by that patient.'

Trusting your team

It is vital that you like and trust your surgeon. If you don't, you can ask for a different one. I did. Remember the doctor who told me I probably had cancer with not a shred of empathy? And the one who didn't explain what 'triple negative' meant when I asked him? Well, those two men were my surgeons initially. And I thought, as an NHS patient, I had no choice in the matter. But then a school-run mum friend, who had also received a breast cancer diagnosis from the same surgeon, told me that she had requested someone different and it was fine. So I googled breast surgeons within my local health trust, found one I liked the look of – the only woman on the list, which appealed to me – and asked if my surgical care could be switched over to her. This was all still on the NHS, and all it took was one call to the breast nurse. It was no big deal at all. It's really important that you feel comfortable with the person who's going to have their hand on the scalpel so, if you're unhappy with your surgeon, please don't hesitate to make a change. As with so many steps in this process, you have to learn to be your own advocate.

So, ideally, you have a surgeon that you trust and can ask anything. This is important because, during my cancer treatment, I became frustrated and upset about never knowing what was around the corner. I was told by one oncologist that my treatment would be finished after mastectomy surgery, only to learn that I was always going to need radiotherapy, since there was cancer in my lymph nodes. And, after radiotherapy, I was put on further chemo to reduce the risk of recurrence. So a treatment programme that I initially hoped would be done and dusted within seven or eight months turned out to take a year and a half. I felt like the goalposts were constantly being moved, and sometimes I felt trapped in a Kafkaesque cycle of endless drugs and tests and radiation and surgery.

When I told my surgeon how I felt, she revealed that doctors sometimes withhold information that isn't immediately relevant, preferring to drip-feed it so that the patient won't feel overwhelmed too early on. I almost exploded: *Why* would they do that? Surely patients deserve to know everything about what they're going to have to go through?

After I had simmered down and was more capable of logical thinking, I realised that not everyone is like me. Many people actually do prefer to know only about the next thing they have to deal with. So, before you meet with your surgeon to discuss your treatment, have a think about what kind of person you are. How much detailed information do you actually want? Do you feel the need to know how long the entire process is going to be, in the worst-case scenario? Because, if you do, you need to be clear in asking exactly what your pathway will look like. You can always change your mind, too. Perhaps initially, you can't think beyond the first tests or the first cycle of chemotherapy. Then, once you're in the swing of treatment, you might want to know more about what's ahead.

Many people want to ask about their prognosis. I certainly did. I wanted numbers and statistics about how many women of my age, with my grade, stage and type of cancer, lived a healthy life after treatment. And precisely how many of them had recurrence. Every doctor is different, and mine (both surgeons and oncologists) were reluctant to talk to me about specific percentages. Through my own research, I discovered the NHS Predict breast cancer online tool, into which you can put details about your own diagnosis and get very specific stats. I quickly wished I hadn't. The results showed that 39 per cent of people with my diagnosis at my age would be dead within five years, 51 per cent dead in 10 years, and 66 per cent dead in 15 years.

Looking back, what was I planning to do with that information? None of us has a one hundred per cent chance of surviving the next five years. Even with perfect health, we might be hit by a bus. The stats for triple negative breast cancer are comparatively bleak, but they are improving all the time and there is still every chance that I'll live a long, cancer-free life. All that information did for me, really, was cause a run of 4 a.m. panic attacks.

So think about *why* you're asking. If it's about you finding it difficult to confront your own mortality, then maybe that's what you need to talk about, whether that be with friends, family, support groups or a professional. Either way, understand that dwelling on the worst-case scenario statistics is not going to get you into the mindset that will help you best cope with treatment. And, yes, I am trying to avoid the dreaded phrase 'stay positive' here. But let's just say that, from experience, I know staying negative is not in your best interest.

Your oncologist

Whatever shape your treatment plan takes, the next person you're likely to meet is your oncologist. They are in charge of all of your non-surgical treatment, whether that be chemotherapy, radiotherapy, hormone therapy or targeted treatments. You might meet different oncologists throughout your treatment because, for example, a medical oncologist can prescribe and manage much of your treatment, but a clinical oncologist is necessary to talk through radiotherapy, if required. Either way, your oncological team should feel cohesive, and each of them ought to be able to explain every step of your treatment plan, if you ask them to.

This is where things start to get complicated because, while surgery is clearly also complex, the concept of it is incredibly simple: they are cutting the cancer out of your body. When you meet your oncologist, you will learn a lot in a short amount of time about various treatments that, unless you have already been through this with someone close to you, you'll probably never have heard of before. It can feel overwhelming and urgent, so it might surprise you to learn that the important thing now is to take a moment. Pause, breathe and think: you almost definitely don't have to rush into anything right away.

Doctor's orders: take your time

Professor Peter Schmid is an internationally renowned breast cancer oncologist. He is clinical director of the Breast Cancer Centre at St Bartholomew's Hospital, and chair in cancer medicine at Barts Cancer Institute, Queen Mary University London.

'A cancer diagnosis is a massive shock, your world is turned upside down,' he says 'Many people's instant reaction is to do something about it as quickly as possible. That's a very natural reaction, but my advice would be to take a step back because, with breast cancer, it is practically never a situation where the decision has to be made at that very moment. It's critical that patients take time to reflect on the information that they have been given, to fully understand the situation. Understand the type of cancer, the treatment options, the functions of the different team members, and the multidisciplinary plan.'

This simply means how all the different elements of treatment work together, and ensuring that your surgeon and oncologist have agreed on what the next year, and beyond, will look like for you.

He explains that it really isn't necessary to rush into anything because, for the majority of patients with primary breast cancer, the outlook is actually very good. The treatments are effective, and there are often options, so make sure you're going into a process that is right for you.

Professor Schmid goes on to compare breast cancer treatment to buying a washing machine, but bear with him because it does actually make sense. 'You look at a washing machine, but then you go away, you think about it, you read reviews, or most of us do,' he says. 'And then you make up your mind after a day or two. But when it comes to cancer, people feel so under pressure and they don't actually take that moment for reflection.'

People even worry that they're going to cause offence by saying that they want time to think about it, he adds, because it might seem as though they are not trusting their medical team. 'But there is a lot of information to digest and it needs to be analysed so you can consider whether this is the right thing for you,' he explains. 'Ideally, patients should have a clear multidisciplinary plan from the beginning because we are all aware of situations where you meet one member of the team, and then get a different view from another member of the team.'

I personally found this to be an issue during treatment because, perhaps since I was being treated at such a large hospital, I rarely met the same person at appointments. And, while the treatment plan didn't vary wildly, I did hear different options, statistics and priorities from different people. In an ideal world, I would have liked to have had more continuity.

When Professor Schmid talks about your multidisciplinary plan, he's referring to the fact that only a small number of patients will receive only one type of treatment. The vast majority of people with a breast cancer diagnosis will require more than one modality, whether that's surgery, radiotherapy, hormone therapy, chemotherapy, targeted treatments or supportive therapy, like bisphosphonates, a group of drugs that slow down bone loss after cancer treatment. It's not only all the different elements of those treatments that you need to be aware of but also the interplay between them.

'I'm always keen to know the plan from the beginning to the

end, which we often can do,' says Professor Schmid. 'And I would like to avoid having to change the plan because it hasn't been mapped out well enough.'

So don't feel uncomfortable about asking to have every step explained in simple terms, and definitely don't worry if the description of your cancer treatment initially sounds like absolute gobbledegook. The various drugs about which you might hear all have such ridiculously convoluted names that, for the first few weeks of treatment, people would ask what kind of chemo I was on and I'd have no idea. It just seemed to be a jumble of unrelated letters that my brain simply couldn't retain. And writing them down makes me feel anxious about narrating the audio version of this book, because I won't be able to pronounce any of them. So that's something to look forward to when we get to the chemotherapy chapter.

A second opinion

Many cases are straightforward and the treatment options will be clear cut. But, if you don't feel one hundred per cent convinced after speaking with your oncologist and surgeon, you can always ask for a second opinion. This doesn't mean that one doctor is wrong and the other is right; it's about helping you to find what's right for you.

'I'm a great advocate of second opinions and I always suggest to my patients that they get one, if they feel they need one,' says Professor Schmid. 'We can only win, as long as you go to an established centre and get a trusted opinion. If they confirm what I said, then the patient will be happier with the treatment plan. If they have more confidence in the decisions I've made, they will ultimately do better psychologically. And, if it's a situation where one of our colleagues comes up with a better idea, then great. We can only benefit from that. It's not very common that someone would come up with a totally different idea, but there is nothing to lose.'

Within the NHS, realistically, it wouldn't be possible to deliver a second opinion for every single patient, but not every patient needs one. There are some breast cancer diagnoses that are well established and others, such as larger triple negative tumours, where newer treatments have been developed more recently.

As you'll realise from reading this book (and as I certainly became aware of from trying to draw all of the best information together into a cohesive and coherent guide), the world of cancer treatment is sprawling and confusing. So, if your oncologist has focused only on the basics during your appointment, you have every right to ask for more information about how it all works and what other options are available.

Please bear in mind that it's different for everyone, and some people appear to breeze through chemotherapy with very few side effects compared to others. But it's good to know what you might have to deal with, and it's important to know that you can *always* talk to your oncologist about whatever it is. Please don't ever feel guilty or that your concern is too small to bother them with. My case was serious in terms of the type and grade of breast cancer, but I was lucky to be receiving curative treatment with the aim of being cancer-free. I felt keenly aware that the oncologists were also dealing with people whose cancer was incurable, who were suffering much more than I was, and who were perhaps running out of options. It made me feel a bit embarrassed to ask if there was anything I could do about my chemo-induced mouth ulcers. But they have the information at their fingertips and can often ease your symptoms in a heartbeat.

Your breast care nurse

This person is a key part of your multidisciplinary team, and will usually be in the room for those important early appointments. She (and they are almost always female; I'm yet to meet a male one, anyway) should have an idea of your overall treatment plan, and where you are in it. If you're wondering what she might be able to help you out with, the short answer is: anything. Your breast care nurse is the link between you and the rest of the medical team. They're your first port of call for everything from physio referrals to finding a post-surgery bra. It will be them who hands you a folder full of leaflets when you are first diagnosed. This pile of reading will seem overwhelming at first, and you probably won't give it much more than a cursory glance initially. But, once you're in the throes of treatment, you'll realise that some of those leaflets actually contain really useful information.

Your breast care nurse will also be able to advise you on concerns, including chemo side effects, in between your oncology appointments. You should be able to get hold of them whenever you need to. In some cases, this can be a bit tricky. You'll have a phone number that will almost always go to voicemail, and you might not always get a call back. I've certainly been in a situation where I've felt cut adrift having left messages on the nurses' answerphone and not been called back. Please don't take this personally; they are notoriously overworked and understaffed. But, when you do get hold of them, you will generally find them to be wonderful and useful. Don't feel uncomfortable about asking them whatever you need to. Of course they're busy, but they're also kind and patient people who will be happy to explain that, yes, your anti-sickness pills do cause constipation, and this is what you can do about it.

'I can't speak for every breast care nurse but, having done that for a long time, I don't think anyone would ever feel you were wasting their time,' says Sally Kum, Breast Cancer Now's associate director of nursing. 'You can ask any question you feel you need to, as every person's concerns are individualised to them. I am asked questions such as "Am I going to die?" as well as practical concerns such as "Can I still drive?"'

They can also signpost you to support outside your medical team. For example, if you're worried you might have lymphoedema (*see page 109*) after surgery to remove your lymph nodes, then they can arrange for you to be assessed and referred – you don't need your doctor to coordinate all your treatment. If you're struggling emotionally, they can refer you to a cancer-specialist psychologist. If you need financial support, they can point you in the direction of the right person at organisations like Macmillan, who provide detailed information about what benefits you might be entitled to, and also grants to pay for things like travel to and from hospital, or even post-surgery bras. I only realised that chemotherapy patients could have the London Congestion Charge reimbursed when I overheard someone else asking for a form at the chemo reception desk (at £15 a day, this was big news). This kind of information is not always easy to come by, or even, as you might assume, automatically dispensed to patients. The breast care nurses should be helping you out with that, because part of their role is to advocate for you, whatever you need.

When I was briskly informed by a male surgeon that there was a 95 per cent chance that the lump in my right breast was cancer, it was a breast care nurse who took me into a room, gave me a tissue, and explained exactly how he'd reached that conclusion. It didn't change the outcome – I still knew the biopsy was likely to result in bad news – but it helped me understand and made me feel cared for during a stressful time.

There may be times when, for whatever reason, you want to speak to somebody outside your medical team. In those instances, there are freephone helplines such as the one run by Breast Cancer Now, which is staffed by breast care nurses. 'Anyone at any stage in their pathway can call that helpline,' says Sally. 'We get calls from people who have a breast symptom and don't know what to do about it, or people who've been referred and are feeling a lot of anxiety and uncertainty. Then we talk to people about their diagnosis, and the types of treatments they're having. Some people call with questions between appointments, things they just didn't think of on the day.'

If you're finding it too hard to pick up the phone, or can't actually speak without crying, then you can also email the Breast Cancer Now nursing team. I love this service, because sometimes you just want to see the information in black and white. And the response is always an in-depth email with links to information or services that might help you. It is rarely possible to email your doctor or breast care nurse in the same way.

If you'd rather speak to someone face to face, then find out about your nearest Maggie's centre or Macmillan Cancer Centre, which are usually situated conveniently on hospital grounds. You can walk in any time, without the need for an appointment, and they will always be happy to help. See the Resources section at the end of the book for contact details of these organisations and more.

DECODING YOUR HOSPITAL LETTERS

Correspondence from your doctor can initially look like a meaningless jumble of letters, but it simply reveals that the medical profession loves an acronym more than most of us.

- IDC = invasive ductal carcinoma
- BI-RADS = breast imaging reporting and data system
- G 1–3 = the cancer's grade, so G3 is grade three
- NMBS = nuclear medicine bone scan
- ALNC = axillary lymph node clearance
- NKDA = no known drug allergies
- SACT = Systemic Anti Cancer Therapy Dataset, the national collection of all cancer chemotherapy data for the NHS in England
- PS 0–4 = PS stands for performance status, and the number shows how much support you need. PS0 means you're active, and PS4 means completely bedridden, with PS1–3 representing a sliding scale in between.

Your Home Support Team

Do not underestimate the importance of those closest to you when you're going through treatment. To me, they were as important as anyone on my medical team. From long, tearful walks with friends, to meals left on my doorstep, to the innumerable ways in which Jonathan helped me when I was at my lowest ebb – lean on your friends and family. Don't ever feel that you have to go through this alone. If you need childcare, or shopping, or just distracting with some gossip, they will honestly be happy to help in any way they can, because it's easy to feel helpless when someone that you care about is going through cancer treatment.

Something that many people find surprising about having cancer though, is how exhausting it can be telling those that love you. This is particularly the case if you are used to being the strongest, most practical or positive person in your family or friendship group. They will be shocked, sad and anxious – of course they will. But often you'll find yourself calming and reassuring people about your own cancer diagnosis, or having to listen as they tell you it's going to be okay (when they can't possibly know that) or 'You've got this', which I heard a lot. It comes from a place of love and kindness, but it's not always helpful.

It's possible that some (potentially very good) friends are less helpful to you than others, and might drain your resources, even though they mean well. A cancer diagnosis can feel as though it's suddenly open season for a wide range of well-meaning friends to ask some seriously personal questions about your body, your fertility, your prognosis and your mental health. It can feel deeply exposing and personal. You might find yourself giving away too much and feeling uncomfortable, or not wanting to answer and feeling rudely evasive. If that's how they make you feel, it's fair to limit or set boundaries on that contact until you feel able to let them back in. Not all friends are created equally and that's absolutely okay. On the other side of the coin are the friends who you might previously have considered less close, who come out of the shadows and absolutely unexpectedly show up for you in the best of ways, right when you need it.

The language of cancer

Some people with a cancer diagnosis can't stand the language that's often used. You might hear people describe you as facing a cancer 'battle' – as if those that have died from cancer simply didn't 'fight' hard enough. I certainly had people telling me that I was 'brave' for sharing so much of my cancer journey on Instagram and through my newspaper columns (side note: some people hate the word 'journey'), which felt wrong to me because I don't think those who choose not to share their experience are any less brave. Also, bravery suggests an element of choice, and none of us is sitting in that chemo chair out of choice.

The other thing that people unintentionally do is minimise your experience. Telling you to 'think positive' feels like an innocuously supportive remark. But, when you're dealing with the shock, fear and uncertainty of a cancer diagnosis, that kind of casual comment can make you feel as though you're failing because you're scared, or even just not a hundred per cent positive all of the time. It doesn't leave room for you to accept that it's perfectly normal to have deep fears about your treatment and beyond. Squashing those fears won't make them go away. They will simply pop up again where you're least expecting them like a particularly grim game of Whac-a-Mole.

Then there are those that try to reassure you with confident claims that breast cancer is 'the best kind' of cancer to get, and one of the most curable. That's true, to an extent. But it remains true that, if breast cancer metastasises (or spreads) elsewhere in the body, it's deadly. Metastatic breast cancer is the biggest killer of women under 50 in the UK, and is second only to Covid in the most recent stats for older women, with 32 women a day dying of it. The people spouting statistics about breast cancer not being that much of a big deal think they're helping you, but minimising your fear is not helpful.

Oddly, I found the most difficult comments to cope with were the ones about my appearance, such as a casual 'It'll grow back' when I was feeling such a sense of dread about losing my hair. Or the absolutely astonishing remark that breast cancer surgery is 'a free boob job'. Women with breast cancer can find this kind of comment most upsetting because they are often struggling with the emotional complexities of appearance that are tied to femininity and identity, and the feeling that it's vain and superficial to feel that way. This is something else that I will address fully later in the book.

People absolutely mean well, so a certain amount of patience and tolerance is required. It's usually easier to nod and smile, unless you know the person well enough to tell them that, actually, you'd prefer it if they didn't describe your experience in that way.

If you have peripheral friends or extended family who often send messages simply asking: 'How are you?' then don't feel bad about having a standard reply saved in the Notes app in your phone that you can simply copy and paste. Something like: 'Queasy and exhausted but hanging in there' is fine. Or simply: 'There are good days and bad days.' They will completely understand if you don't reply at all but, if you're a people pleaser like I am, then it can be quite un-relaxing to have messages to which you haven't replied in your WhatsApp. You might become very aware of your limits when struggling with fatigue during cancer treatment, and find that you have to choose carefully where you put your energy. If you're spending all your emotional energy in replying to messages from colleagues and acquaintances, at the expense of playing with your kids, for instance, then you have to reassess the situation. My favourite kind of message was always one that simply said: 'I'm thinking of you and sending love, no need to reply.'

With close friends and family that you live with, or that you see more often, you're going to have to be honest about what you want, because they won't know unless you tell them. Jonathan can attest that I've snapped at him for trying to look for solutions or ways to 'fix' the situation when I was upset. When, often, all I needed was someone to listen, and to be there with me in the misery while I cried it out.

Find your tribe

You might find it difficult to talk honestly to those closest to you about how you're feeling, and that's really common. You're probably painfully aware that your partner, parent or close friend already finds it hard to see someone they love go through something as bleak and gruelling as cancer treatment. They can tend to overly reassure or try to distract you, because all they want is to see you smile. And that isn't always a terrible idea; it certainly has its place. During chemo, Jonathan and I had 'romcom Fridays', where every week we'd watch a classic romantic comedy, from *When Harry Met Sally* to *How to Lose a Guy in 10 Days*. He understood that sometimes I just needed to switch my brain off and laugh at the tribulations of beautiful people awkwardly falling in love.

Meanwhile, I've had friends hastily try to change the subject when they see that talking about hair loss or mastectomy surgery is making me tearful. If you want to have a good old cry, then tell them that. If you want to be distracted and think about anything but cancer, then also tell them. They will appreciate the guidance, because it's hard for people to know what to say when you're going through something they know is horrific, but they don't fully understand it.

This is where it can be extremely helpful to find people who *do* understand what you're going through. Much like your NCT friends are vital on maternity leave, when you can't talk to your childfree mates about whether or not your baby's poo looks normal, finding your breast cancer tribe can make all the difference. Social media is great for this; I found people on Instagram who are now friends for life, simply because we were going through cancer treatment at the same time. Your cancer community might form more organically if there is another mum at the school gate, colleague at work or acquaintance in your yoga class who has been through the same thing.

Organisations like Macmillan, Maggie's and Future Dreams also run support groups and drop-in coffee mornings where you can meet other people with breast cancer. Initially, you might feel as though you don't need external support. I strongly felt that I had good friends and a close family, and they would be all I needed. There was also a nagging sense for me that seeking more help would be 'giving in' to my unwanted identity as a 'cancer person'. Clearly, that was ridiculous, and I eventually realised that it was a huge support to speak to other women who truly understood what I was going through. Also, your exhaustion and anxiety is a lot to place on someone else's shoulders, particularly when they feel powerless to help. I'm not saying don't talk to those closest to you about how you're feeling – you definitely should do that – I just mean that it's good to have other people onto whom you can offload your most fraught emotions, as well. Particularly if they include an expert who is up to speed on the latest information and research relevant to you.

Play it by ear and do what feels right. You don't have to sign up to the first support group you hear about. I did initially, and attended one that was online (obviously, because of the pandemic), and found it an unbelievably depressing line-up of people complaining about their litany of grim side effects and emotions. Eventually I wrote something in the chat about having to get to an appointment and left the Zoom. On the other hand, I have been to events at Future Dreams House, a dedicated breast cancer support centre in King's Cross, which felt positive, galvanising and inspiring. It's about finding what works for you.

Breast Cancer Now has initiatives such as Someone Like Me, where you can email or speak to a volunteer who has been through cancer treatment. This is particularly helpful if your cancer is not one of the most common types, or if you are a man, because you can speak to someone who knows exactly how you feel. There is a monthly virtual meet-up for men with breast cancer, supported by a number of charities, including Walk the Walk and the Male Breast Cancer Coalition (MBCC). Find it online, and do speak to someone, because there can be fewer opportunities for men to talk about their experience.

Another one of Breast Cancer Now's groups is called Younger Women Together, for those under 45 to talk about issues such as fertility, body image and returning to work. 'The overwhelming feedback from our younger women's groups is that people really do value the power of that peer-to-peer discussion, that shared experience,' says Sally Kum of Breast Cancer Now. 'But also the nurses get lots of patients saying, "My friendship group is really tight, but they don't know what to say." So we would advise friends of someone with breast cancer to actually ask them what they want. Some people don't want to think about cancer every day: they want to go away, forget that they've got cancer, and have fun with their friends. Then, on other days, they might want to have those discussions or show you what their scars look like so that you can try and empathise with where they're coming from.'

One thing's for sure, you will need people to talk to, so do identify those in your life who are good listeners. They acknowledge that what you're going through is horrendous, they validate your feelings and allow you to vent when you need to. Treasure those people, and learn from them, because one day you will very likely need to be that person for someone else.

Your rights at work

Now that breast cancer is affecting more younger women, more and more of us are having to consider what we do about work, on top of all the other decisions to make around cancer treatment. Ideally, your workplace and immediate boss will be kind and understanding, giving you as much time off as you need. However, some people might feel that they are no longer able to continue in their current role, and others may be self-employed and dealing with the financial hardship that comes with inevitably reduced hours.

It's difficult for me to give specific advice around this, since everyone's situation is so different. But if you're reading this and panicking about money during cancer treatment, please get in touch with Macmillan Cancer Support right away. They have lots of advice and resources about what benefits you are entitled to, and other ways in which you can get financial support during this time. They will even fill out as much of the statutory sick pay forms for you as they can, asking you to do only the bare minimum. The importance of this cannot be overstated when you're overwhelmed, dealing with brain fog, and realising that the admin around cancer treatment can feel like a full-time job, for which you are woefully ill-prepared.

How can I help?

People often ask this question, which is very kind. But it does rather put the onus on you to come up with something, on top of everything else you have to think about. So here's a handy cut-out-and-keep list of practical ways to help. You could pick one idea, use this list to inspire another or simply take a picture of this page and send it to them. They want to help, after all. So let them.

1. It's exhausting to plan meals during cancer treatment, so a dish left on the doorstep is always appreciated. Or vouchers for a healthy ready-meal company like Cook.
2. It's useful to have someone who is able to be on call to pick up the kids from school, collect prescriptions, help with lifts to hospital or just sit with you during chemo.
3. Good listeners are always needed. Sometimes you want to vent your sadness and/or anger to someone who can listen without trying to 'fix' things.
4. Having said that, sometimes you want to forget about cancer and have a laugh. Could they arrange to watch a fun film, or just turn up with some juicy gossip?
5. In terms of gifts, think practical mood-boosters, like cashmere socks, a nice moisturiser, posh pyjamas or bath salts. Not flowers please, unless there is a person around who will reliably put them in a vase, keep the water topped up and throw them out when they die.
6. Talking of which, don't forget about the person who is the main support for the person with cancer, whether that's a partner, parent, friend or offspring. They need support, too.

Embracing Acceptance

I learned early on that it's counterproductive to sit around wishing you didn't have cancer. That doesn't mean it's easy to accept your diagnosis. It's hard, and it will look different for everybody because there is no 'doing it right'.

But acceptance is a really important step in moving forward. It doesn't mean being totally fine with having cancer, sugar-coating your experience, or expecting yourself to just get on with your daily activities no matter how distraught you might be feeling. In fact, feeling all of the feelings is vital for acceptance, so it's really helpful to find a way to express your grief at diagnosis. Because it *is* a form of grief: for your pre-surgery body, your pre-cancer identity and comparatively carefree life. Trust the process, don't rush. Lean into actually 'being ill' and use this time as a moment to slow everything right down to the essentials.

Early on in your diagnosis, it's a whirlwind. You are rushed from scan to test to treatment to appointment, with an ever-growing pile of cancer admin to attend to. Appointment times change, your medications vary depending on your side effects and how you're responding to treatment, and, if your cancer clinic is anything like mine, it's a different oncologist every time you go, so there isn't even the reassuring continuity of a familiar face. But try and carve out some time to consider what this all means for you; how you feel about stepping back from the day-to-day stuff that felt so important before your cancer diagnosis.

Some people find meditation useful as a tool for checking in with themselves. Others find it impossible to sit with their own thoughts during a time of enormous disruption. If that's the case, then you might find it easier to talk it through.

In the previous chapter, I ran through the options for connecting with other women going through breast cancer treatment, either online or in person at places like Maggie's. But, of course, you can always seek professional counselling if you feel that might help you. If you choose to be referred through the NHS, then talk to your oncologist rather than your GP, because not only might they be able to fast-track the process but they may well also have access to a therapist who specialises in dealing with cancer patients. The other option is to seek therapy privately, which will be quicker to access, with the added benefit that you can ask your local friends for a recommendation. Therapists are a bit like building contractors: you can't know how good they are until you're actually working together, so it's usually advisable to get a recommendation rather than take a shot in the dark.

Accepting non-productivity

Dr Lisa Dvorjetz is a counselling psychologist who has worked with cancer patients through the East London and Royal Marsden NHS Foundation Trusts. She tells me that, in her experience, women can even feel as if they are to blame for the ways in which their diagnosis is affecting those closest to them. If that sounds ridiculous and irrational, you'd be amazed at how common it is.

'Very often patients feel guilty if they aren't doing what they used to, especially in a society that places a high value on productivity and achievements in life,' she explains. 'For example, not being able to work due to fatigue or being unable to physically cope with the same number of tasks as before the cancer. This, in turn, makes people feel that they are letting others down, being a burden, feeling useless, and generally having critical thoughts towards themselves.'

Cancer treatment makes this particularly hard because everybody is different in their response to it. Some people appear to manage chemo with barely any side effects, whereas others are so wracked with fatigue they can't get out of bed for weeks. Most likely, you will have days where you feel capable of working and socialising, and days when you can barely walk around the block, but the uncertainty about how you're going to feel from day to day can be emotionally exhausting and make it difficult to plan ahead. The best approach is to remove as much pressure as possible by clearing your calendar and focusing fully on rest and recuperation, only adding in things at the last minute if you're up to it. If at all possible, taking time out from work, social and family commitments is not just a feel-good suggestion, but, says Dr Dvorjetz, it's essential to maintaining psychological balance. This may mean that you need to accept the guilt, in order to prioritise rest.

Accepting fear

Of course, there's another big feeling to accept, and it's one that is front and centre of most people's minds from the moment they receive a cancer diagnosis: fear. This is one of the biggest barriers for people in coming to terms with their diagnosis, explains Dr Dvorjetz. 'Many people say they don't want to think about cancer because, if they ignore it, then the worrying thoughts and feelings won't surface. But what we know is that the more we actively try not to think about something, the more we end up thinking about it!'

The first step she says, is to acknowledge the feelings of fear or anxiety. 'What are the fearful thoughts that are being experienced? Can you physically feel the fear in your body? Some people describe a tightness in their chest, sweaty palms, or a racing heartbeat. Those are all normal bodily reactions when your body suspects danger and retreats into survival mode.' She suggests breathing techniques as a practical tool to calm down the body's fight-or-flight response and switch off anxious thinking. This regulates the body's nervous system by showing it that there is no imminent physical danger (*see page 54*).

It can be easy to feel as though everyone else is coping, and you're the only one that's falling apart. But, when you meet other women going through treatment for breast cancer or follow them online, you don't see their 4 a.m. panic attacks or them crying in the shower. It's important to be clear that every single person with cancer sometimes feels as though they're falling apart, even if on the outside they seem very much together. Understanding this, and the fact that it's not easy – for anyone – is a key part of coming to terms with your diagnosis.

Acceptance is not about dismissing your valid feelings of fear, anger and sadness, but acknowledging them, while simultaneously helping your nervous system understand that – here and now – you are safe. Embracing fear and sadness in tough times can actually allow us to live more authentically and vividly. This experience could make you a better person, with a greater sense of empathy for what others might be going through and a keener awareness of the fact that life is short, and precious.

And acceptance certainly does not mean being happy, or even being fine, with having cancer. Nobody wants to have cancer, and there's no point pretending otherwise. But, equally, it's not helpful to pretend it's not happening. That will only lead to all those difficult emotions bubbling up after treatment has finished. This is something that is incredibly common, and I'll address it fully later.

Importantly, acceptance is not a destination that you reach, after which you can relax. There will be good days and bad days, ups and downs, probably for ever. But that's life, right? And we're lucky to be living it.

Carly's story

Carly Moosah was 37 when she was diagnosed with breast cancer in December 2019, five months after her big sister had been diagnosed with ovarian cancer (they both later discovered they carry the BRCA1 gene mutation). She describes it as something she had feared for most of her life, since her grandmother and her mother both died of secondary breast cancer. So, when she was diagnosed, she was absolutely terrified.

'Having held my mum's hand as she died just a decade earlier, I knew how this could go,' she says. 'Cancer had cruelly taken the most important person in my life and it felt like it was now coming for me.' At the time, her children were four and six and, for their sakes, if not for her own, she realised she couldn't let crippling fear and anxiety take over her life. She would have to accept the diagnosis to be able to cope with treatment in a pragmatic way, and stop her mind running away with what-ifs.

Knowing how much cancer treatment had developed over the past 10 years, in addition to the fact that her cancer was triple negative while her mum's had been hormonal - which meant her treatment plan was to look very different - Carly was able to separate her mother's story from her own and focus on her own path. 'I needed to detach myself from the disease being a death sentence,' she says. This makes it sound as though she managed to do that easily, but, of course, it was a process requiring emotional tools and conscious effort. In Carly's case, meditation eased her anxiety, and helped her to be more present in each moment. This sense of presence, as well as a conscious choice to focus on gratitude rather than fear, allowed her to look forward in a positive way. She also had therapy and, ironically, learned to find a confidence and acceptance in herself and her body that she hadn't had pre-cancer.

'Facing my own mortality gave me an inner strength that I'm proud of, and a zest for life that I carry with me today,' she says. 'But first I had to let go of how I thought my life would look. Compassion-focused therapy gave me the space to process everything that I was feeling. Letting go is never easy but, ultimately, holding onto the person I was before cancer was only adding to my grief. Once I drew that line in the sand, I found a sense of peace and knowing that everything is as it has to be. I wouldn't be who I am today without cancer. Do I wish it had never had to happen? Of course. But do I embrace who I am because of it? Absolutely.'

This transformative process isn't easy but, as Carly has shown, it is possible. It takes time though. Carly advises really taking the time to feel sad about saying goodbye to the person you were before cancer treatment. People often talk about wanting their old self back after breast cancer, but it isn't possible to go back to exactly how you were before. So mourn for the person you were, allowing yourself the space to really feel all of those difficult feelings, before moving forward in a more positive way. How this looks will be different for everyone, in the same way that grief is different for everyone. Give in to the sadness of losing the old you. Then, Carly says, you need to find your support system – whether that's therapy or a support group – and identify your emotional reinforcements.

'There are so many people out there who have been carrying the cancer baton and, although it might feel as though it has been passed to you to run along solo, we are all there running alongside you,' Carly insists. 'You are not alone. We're cheering you on, and we're here to pick you up when you fall. It is said so often that cancer is the worst club to become a member of, but I'll shout from the rooftops that once in, it has the most epic members of all time.'

And, she says, cancer doesn't only take away. 'Cancer took so much from me but, ultimately, it gave me a huge lease of life. I was looking at the world through a hazy lens before my diagnosis, thinking that I had all the time in the world. This experience made me realise with crystal clarity that I don't know how long I have but, whatever time I do have, I want to spend it nourishing myself, enjoying the small moments, and connecting with people that make me feel good. Cancer gave me that.'

TOOLS FOR ACCEPTANCE

- Meditation and mindfulness. There are plenty of free online resources to help with this.
- Professional counselling. Ask to be referred through your breast care nurse, or look into private options, which will likely be quicker to access.
- Hypnosis works wonders for some people, although you have to be open to the process.
- Identify your support system: the friends and family that won't pressure you into being your old self again, and will instead sit with you through the hard feelings, and be there on the other side.
- Box breathing. Visualise the four sides of a square, then inhale deeply for four counts, hold your breath four counts, exhale for four counts and, again, hold for four counts. Imagine each of those steps as one of the sides of the square, and follow them round as you go. The visualisation gives your mind something soothing to focus on, and prevents spiralling thoughts. Repeat that pattern of breathing for at least a minute, ideally two. This technique has been shown scientifically to soothe the nervous system.

- Small wins. This could be anything from going for a walk with a friend, to having a bath and doing some kind of skincare routine. Making an effort to find time to do things like that, and ticking them off as something you have achieved, makes a huge difference. People dismiss ideas like being outside in nature or doing yoga as airy-fairy self-care nonsense, but the cumulative impact of these small actions is bigger than you think.

An Integrated Approach to Cancer Treatment

Cancer patients (and people, generally) can tend to split into two camps. There are those who accept every treatment their doctor recommends and believe lifestyle advice is superfluous to medical oncology. Then there are those who shudder at the toxic nature of cancer treatment, and believe they can shrink tumours only with a combination of positive thinking and kale.

As with most things in life, I believe the truth is somewhere in the middle. I trust in science, and underwent every treatment that my oncologist advised, including brutal AC chemo and Taxol/Carbo (*see page 120*), followed by mastectomy surgery, radiotherapy and capecitabine, taken as adjuvant chemo. But I also strongly believe – and science supports this – that what you eat, drink, think and do can hugely impact the severity of side effects, the efficacy of your treatment and the risk of recurrence.

But, unless you get lucky, NHS doctors are unlikely to recommend lifestyle medicine, or even mention it. I know this from personal experience, going back 15 years before I had cancer. When I was 25, I went to the doctor because my periods had become increasingly sporadic. After a series of tests, I was diagnosed with polycystic ovary syndrome and prescribed a drug called metformin. The endocrinologist said PCOS is a chronic condition so I'd be on medication for life. I didn't like the idea of that, so I did my own research and learned that PCOS is related to insulin resistance and metformin works by regulating your blood sugar. So I changed my diet. This was the era when low-carb diets like Atkins and the GI diet were really popular, although, until then, I had paid them little attention since I didn't feel the need to lose weight. I started reading about how to reduce blood sugar spikes, and doing things like sipping apple cider vinegar before meals and paying attention to the fibre in my carbs. At 25, I was not the healthiest eater, but I tried to lower the glycaemic load of my less-healthy choices by having, for example, hummus with my crisps and nuts with my chocolate. Over several weeks, I weaned myself off the metformin. At a follow-up appointment, I told the endocrinologist what I'd done, and said my periods were back to normal so I didn't need any more medication. 'That's great,' he exclaimed. 'You've fixed it through lifestyle.'

I left feeling pretty pleased with myself, but wondering why the NHS hadn't told me that I could do that? Surely it's better to explain a simple lifestyle fix than to pay for someone to be on medication for life? Why did I have to work it out for myself? I guess, if you asked a doctor, they'd say that they're over-stretched and have very little time with patients. Also, they may feel that people can be trusted to take a pill, but not to make changes to their diet and stick to it long-term. Sadly, this means, as patients, we often can't trust doctors to provide simple lifestyle advice that could mean fewer drugs, and therefore fewer side effects.

To be clear, I'm absolutely not saying that lifestyle changes can replace chemo or cure cancer. But the litany of drugs that are prescribed around chemo could surely be reduced: anti-sickness pills, plus laxatives to combat the constipation that's a side effect of the anti-sickness pills; steroids, plus sleeping pills to combat the wired-but-tired effect of the steroids. Even codeine for mouth ulcers. There is a culture of over-treatment, especially for younger patients whose bodies can tolerate it. And, at the time, I didn't even consider that I didn't have to accept *every* treatment that was offered to me.

I didn't know anything about integrative oncology when I started cancer treatment, but I knew that the sheer volume of drugs I was imbibing was having a negative effect on my physiology. To the extent that, towards the end of chemo, I had instinctively reduced them. I made fresh ginger tea to reduce sickness, and stopped taking the anti-sickness pills. I also slowly reduced the steroid dose. And, I'm slightly ashamed to admit this now, I did it without telling my oncologist because I almost felt I'd be in trouble for not taking all the drugs. The truth is, my oncologist would probably have been open to a conversation about other ways of managing side effects.

The drugs are there if you need them, but you do have options, and choosing to support yourself through cancer treatment in other ways does not mean rejecting conventional medicine, at all.

What is integrative treatment?

Integrative cancer care is not about dismissing doctors' advice or going all-or-nothing into some alternative therapy or other. It simply means using other techniques alongside your medical treatment, to assuage anxiety, counteract the toxicity of chemo and put you in the best place to cope with treatment and reduce your risk of recurrence. Win-win, right?

But many are resistant to the idea – which is why I was fearful of talking about it at the time – and I get why. There is a disturbing number of weird and wacky treatments, diets and supplements available, which claim to cure or prevent cancer. And unfortunately there are people out there peddling expensive but unnecessary products and therapies, and taking advantage of desperate and vulnerable cancer patients.

One way to discern quackery from a good source of information is to dismiss anything offering a wonder cure, or using the phrase 'prevent' cancer. Any proper expert will tell you there is no way that any one drug, food, supplement or tonic can prevent cancer, since the causes of cancer are so varied. The best claim that anyone can make would be to 'reduce your risk', which doesn't sound as sexy.

And the things that have been proven to reduce your risk are the things that don't require you to fork out much money. It's things like exercise, good nutrition, stress management and sleep. Because in reality, there is no silver bullet. You need to take into account your whole lifestyle. If you have a sedentary life, with a lot of stress, too little sleep and a reliance on processed convenience foods, you can't expect a supplement to make much difference. It's about a web of interconnected elements: how you eat, move, sleep and connect with the things that matter to you. I know that sounds like hard work, but lifestyle change in one area of your life always positively impacts the others. For example, cutting down on alcohol reduces hangover-fuelled binge eating. And getting more restorative sleep helps you feel calmer and more focused at work, as well as giving you the energy to move your body more throughout the day.

It is simple steps like this that are known as lifestyle medicine or, in cancer terms, 'integrative oncology'. The British Society for Integrative Oncology describes it as: 'A patient-centred, evidence-informed field of cancer care that utilises nutritional, lifestyle and complementary interventions alongside conventional cancer treatments to support better quality of life, improve resilience, minimise the side effects of treatment and improve outcomes.'

If the phrase 'complementary interventions' is off-putting, don't worry. No one's going to ask you to imbibe moon dust. It can be as simple as moving your body more. In Australia, for instance, an exercise plan is prescribed along with your medical treatment, because movement is one element of lifestyle medicine that has been scientifically proven to help you better cope with treatment and reduce your risk of recurrence. As a report for the World Economic Forum put it: 'If the effects of exercise could be encapsulated in a pill, it would be prescribed to every cancer patient worldwide and viewed as a major breakthrough in cancer treatment.'[1]

During chemo, I had no energy for exercise, and I thought that was fine. Surely rest was the most important thing? In reality, neglecting moving my body was detrimental to my energy levels and overall health. I wish someone had told me at the time that there are studies showing people who work out during chemotherapy cope better in terms of fatigue levels, nausea, hot flushes and anxiety. It's a significant difference, so it's really worth doing as much as you can manage. I'm not saying you have to drag yourself out of your sickbed and pump iron in the gym. It can be as simple as a walk around the block, a gentle online yoga class, or just a few squats and lunges in your living room. Entirely rejecting movement (a term I prefer to exercise, which suggests scheduled sweat sessions) can lead to deteriorating muscle mass, and can become a vicious circle because it's more difficult to build it back up. As I discovered when I attempted to do a Couch to 5k run soon after finishing chemo, and had to sheepishly stagger home after five minutes.

Other lifestyle interventions have less hard evidence to back them up. A randomised controlled trial works with drugs, but rarely for dietary choices or stress management. Why? First, it would be unethical to do a study where you expose people to something potentially dangerous, such as plying cancer patients with processed food or sugary drinks. And studies that rely on people reporting back on what they've eaten are unreliable, frankly, because people are unreliable. And how do you study stress in a randomised trial? Are you going to put some women in a highly stressful situation? Or some in a completely stress-free environment, as if that's a thing that even exists?

While integrated approaches are already incorporated alongside cancer treatment in countries including Australia and the United States, the NHS is almost uniquely handcuffed with regards to this advice unless it's proven to be definitively curative. It appears the only way to do it is through a generic leaflet that is handed out at diagnosis, and not patient specific.

This is clearly not ideal because what works well for some

people might not work for others. For instance, studies have shown the benefits of acupuncture for cancer patients, in terms of relieving nausea, fatigue, low mood and chronic pain. But, if you're terrified of needles and spend the whole session tensed up in a ball of stress, it probably isn't doing you that much good. Meditation has been found to relieve anxiety and pain in some cancer patients, but others find that sitting alone with their thoughts can cause spiralling fears to engulf them. Some find that practising yoga helps ease their anxiety, fatigue and insomnia. Others just hate yoga, and prefer to sweat it out in their local boxing club. It's about finding what works for you.

COMPLEMENTARY IDEAS

I'm not suggesting you try *all* of these, or even any of them, if none appeal. These are just a few ideas to get you thinking of different ways to support yourself through treatment. The benefits of some of these approaches might be put down to a placebo effect, but a placebo effect is still an effect. And if one of these therapies helps with – for example – stress management or reducing anxiety, then that's an inarguable benefit. Just go into it with realistic expectations.

Acupuncture Fine needles are inserted into the body at specific points that may help support the flow of energy, known as Qi in Traditional Chinese Medicine. Western medical acupuncture is a modern interpretation of this. It has been shown to help with nausea and fatigue, as well as menopausal symptoms like hot flushes.

Reiki A form of energy healing, involving the practitioner putting their hands on or just above your body, which many people find deeply relaxing. It has the benefit of being completely non-invasive so, at the very least, you certainly won't have any negative effects from it.

Reflexology Gentle pressure is applied to your feet during this relaxing treatment that works on energy pathways similar to acupuncture (but without the needles). It is said to be beneficial for everything from stress relief to lymphatic flow, and even constipation.

Yoga There are lots of different types of yoga, but almost all of them can help with improving flexibility and balance, building strength, and soothing your nervous system through breathing techniques.

Homeopathy A homeopath concocts natural remedies in the form of pills, creams or tonics, and you will come across people who swear by them. There are some instances where homeopathic remedies have been shown to have positive effects, such as calendula for inflamed skin or arnica for bruising. But the NHS advises against the remedies for anything more than relaxation or managing stress and anxiety. If you want to try it, I'd suggest doing your research to find a homeopath you trust and getting personalised advice, rather than spending money willy-nilly on random homeopathic remedies.

The science is there

This is a complicated, often controversial, space – but I'm going to help you navigate it with the help of experts who have been studying integrative oncology for decades.

'To me, it means the best of everything,' explains Dr Nina Fuller-Shavel, a precision health and integrative medicine doctor and co-chair of the British Society for Integrative Oncology (BSIO). 'People should have access to the most recent, advanced conventional medicine but, alongside that, we should be looking at nutrition, lifestyle, wellbeing, sleep and evidence-informed complementary therapies. Not just some random stuff, but a proven, targeted, personalised approach.'

And when she says proven, she means the hard evidence is there for many lifestyle interventions. Dr Fuller-Shavel is a medical doctor and scientist with two degrees in Natural Sciences and Medicine from the University of Cambridge. She is not interested in assumptions or wishful thinking, and she points me in the direction of several studies showing the benefits for cancer patients of movement, sleep, good nutrition, and managing stress, anxiety and depression with psycho-emotional support.

Back in 2017, the Society for Integrative Oncology (the US-based organisation that was a precursor to the BSIO) produced clinical guidelines on the safety and benefits of using an integrative approach, based on a systematic review of all the available research. They looked at the benefits in terms of the side effects of many cancer treatments: fatigue, low mood, lymphoedema, peripheral neuropathy, and menopausal symptoms such as hot flushes. In 2018, the guidelines were reviewed by the American Society of Clinical Oncology, which is the leading professional body for oncology in the world. They endorsed the guidelines, which were then published in the prestigious *Journal of Clinical Oncology*. So the science is very much there.

That all makes it sound as though these approaches are now widely understood and implemented. But, unfortunately, it didn't change cancer treatment in the way that you might hope. Most people with breast cancer in the UK are not being offered, or even told about, any of these evidence-based additional tools, even if they're presenting with symptoms or side effects of cancer treatment that integrative approaches have been shown in trials to help.

Why not? Well, as anyone who has spent all afternoon waiting for a delayed hospital appointment knows, British breast clinicians are busy people. And they're not always aware of these guidelines or taught about these approaches in their training, even though they're published in prestigious journals. It just doesn't register because it's not the sort of thing that doctors are trained to be interested in.

'In all of my years of medical training, I had two hours on nutrition, and some doctors don't even get that,' explains Dr Fuller-Shavel. Although, she continues, the lack of basic lifestyle training is not the biggest issue. Rather, it's that we need a mindset shift, away from the idea that, if a doctor doesn't know about it, then it's irrelevant. 'Doctors don't need to be an expert in integrative oncology,' she says. 'But what we do need is a willingness for them to be open and say, "I don't know about this, but I'm going to check with someone who does." At the BSIO, we're very happy to share information and educate oncologists in lifestyle interventions.'

Even if doctors are aware of the benefits, there is little funding within the NHS to deliver integrative services. Where it is available, it's mostly provided by charities or volunteers. If you have private healthcare, you are more likely to be offered the opportunity to try an integrated approach. For example, the Nuffield Health centre at St Bartholomew's Hospital in London encourages their patients to take part in a 12-week cancer rehabilitation programme at the nearby Barbican Fitness and Wellbeing Centre, where specialist physiotherapists and fitness professionals have had specific training in the physical issues stemming from cancer treatment and surgery.

If, like me (and most people in the UK), you are an NHS patient, then your breast care nurse is probably the best person to chat to about such approaches if your oncologist is being less than forthcoming. But even then, they can only really tell you about the things that are available within your specific NHS trust.

Cancer care in the UK generally does not take a holistic approach – as much as you might want your doctor to make these suggestions as the expert in the room, it's unlikely to be something they will offer as a treatment option.

Perhaps because of the dismissive attitude of many medical professionals, studies have shown that most people who use complementary services don't even tell their oncologist about it, for fear of being thought of as a 'difficult' patient. It's the same feeling I had when I kept quiet about reducing my steroid dose.

'We need to have it out in the open, and allow patients to feel comfortable discussing it with their oncologist, because it isn't one-size-fits-all,' says Dr Fuller-Shavel. 'There are studies in the US – where there is more conversation about this sort of thing than we have here in the UK – saying that the number of people actually using complementary therapies is at least a third more than oncologists think it is. And that's a gap that I don't like.'

Complementary, not alternative

To help them be more open to these ideas, and less dismissive, perhaps oncologists and surgeons need to be persuaded that accessing a complementary therapy doesn't mean that patients will abandon their medical treatment plan. In fact, it has been reported that patients are actually more likely to stick with conventional treatment if they have found that an integrative approach helps them better cope with the side effects. Not only will they feel more positive about the outcome, but they will also feel heard and supported. Some people refer to complementary treatments as 'alternative' therapies, which is an unhelpful word because it sounds as though the treatment is an alternative to conventional medicine, which I suppose may sometimes be the case, but not at all in this instance.

'That's such a misconception, because nothing that I do is "alternative" to medical cancer treatment,' says Dr Fuller-Shavel. 'Everybody's under dual care. It has to be a discussion, and you absolutely have choices. You need a team. So there's your medical team in the NHS, then you might need a wider team because your NHS team perhaps does not have all the knowledge. There is also charity support like Penny Brohn UK or Yes to Life. What the BSIO is trying to do now is start educating healthcare professionals as to what are the evidence-based options out there.'

The reason she feels so passionately about this is that her work is based on her own experience. Dr Fuller-Shavel was just 33 when she received her own breast cancer diagnosis. And, from the beginning, she was clear with her medical team that she would not be relying on them for all of her care.

'I had to convince my oncologist and my oncoplastic surgeon, but they could see how well I was progressing during chemotherapy,' she explains. 'They could see the benefits, in terms of quality of life, that they were not seeing in other patients. My prof said to me: "You're like a breath of fresh air in here because everybody's struggling with side effects, but it seems like you're doing something to manage them." That's why I feel so strongly that some of the simplest things we can deliver in terms of nutrition, lifestyle, sleep support and psycho-emotional support should be available on the NHS, perhaps in a group setting,' she continues. 'All three sectors – charity, private and the NHS – need to work together to provide the best of the best, rather than sitting in their separate corners doing their own separate things, because that actually doesn't benefit anybody.'

There is evidence for complementary treatments as wide-ranging as yoga, acupuncture and CBT (cognitive behavioural therapy), as well as nutrition and movement. The aim of many of these approaches is often to support your mental health through cancer treatment but, actually, some follow-up studies have shown that overall physical health can also improve.

Think of a cancerous tumour as a seed in some soil. Oncologists can poison the seed with chemo to destroy it, or they can burn it with radiotherapy, but they don't often pay attention to the soil, which represents everything else about how you live your life. It seems obvious to me that the microenvironment around the cancer can make a big difference as to whether it grows quickly or slowly, or even shrinks. There is evidence that smoking, drinking alcohol and eating ultra-processed foods might provide the kind of soil that will encourage cancer growth. Whereas exercise, a wide range of different coloured fruits and vegetables, as well as good sleep and stress management, will produce the kind of soil that's going to grow healthier cells.

The NHS vs the rest of the world

A quick word in defence of the NHS. It absolutely saved my life, and it was completely free. Yes, it's over-stretched and by no means perfect, but I am incredibly grateful for it. I have mentioned other countries' approach to cancer treatment, including the US where the system is more integrated, but it's important to add that American healthcare is only great if you are well insured.

Carlie Thompson MD is a board-certified and fellowship-trained breast surgical oncologist and assistant professor of surgery at UCLA Health in Los Angeles. On paper, cancer care in the US sounds amazing. 'I reserve a full hour of my clinic time with a newly diagnosed breast cancer patient,' she tells me. 'I go through their medical history and pathology report, really making sure they understand what subtype of breast cancer they have. I talk them through every step of treatment, so they have an idea of what the whole process looks like. I also talk about diet and lifestyle, and how that interacts with everything, particularly with oestrogen-sensitive cancers. Then I am always assessing where patients are at from a psychological perspective, and whether they need any psychological support. Finally, one of my goals of the initial visit is to assess what a woman's relationship is with her breasts, so I can take that into consideration when we're making surgical decisions.'

I think back to the brisk 10-minute appointment at which I learned I had breast cancer. The doctor explained that

I needed to have chemotherapy before surgery, but there was no discussion about what kind of surgery I might have, no mention of radiotherapy, and no sense of how long the whole process would take. It's far-fetched to imagine that he might have made time to talk through things like diet and exercise with me.

Dr Thompson believes these approaches are absolutely vital in cancer treatment and beyond. 'I look at it as attacking the problem from another direction,' she explains. 'It's immensely important. Obviously it's going to depend on the patient and the patient's beliefs around those therapies as well. But, especially for patients where those practices are already a part of their life in some way, it's so important for the support of psychological wellbeing. That's where those practices, like mindfulness strategies and complementary therapies, can really help: with the mind–body connection.'

This is the first time I've heard a doctor mention the mind-body connection (*see also page 105 for more on this*). But Dr Thompson admits that practical advice around diet and lifestyle is 'very provider-specific'. Where she is based, at the UCLA Revlon Breast Clinic in Los Angeles there are dieticians on hand to work with patients who need additional support in that area, in the same way that they might have psychologists available if needed. 'At cancer centres and larger academic institutions, it's very much on our radar,' she says. 'A lot of providers probably don't cover diet and lifestyle, unless the patient directly asks them a question about it, just because there's a lot to talk about at those visits. How much we each spend on that, as individual providers, is going to vary a lot. You might not get that same level of attention to complementary treatment options in smaller centres.'

So while it may feel as though the US is ahead of us in some ways, with integrative cancer care often a part of standard treatment, this is not always the case. Without a system like the NHS, there is a lack of healthcare equity. Health insurance varies wildly, with some providers covering your mastectomy but not your reconstruction. When the actress Julia Louis-Dreyfus was diagnosed with breast cancer in 2017, she used her platform to campaign to raise funds for women whose insurance didn't cover reconstruction. And, if you don't have health insurance at all, then you will be saddled with enormous bills that could leave you debt-ridden for life.

In other countries, access to resources above and beyond the standard treatment appears to be more egalitarian. In Germany, for instance, the system is funded by statutory contributions, ensuring free healthcare for all. As in the UK, you can also take out private health insurance if you want to. But every cancer patient is offered a three-week course of cancer rehab. Mind-blowingly, people stay in a specially designed rehabilitation centre (for three weeks!) and receive physiotherapy, fitness training, occupational therapy, psychological counselling, nutritional information and training in relaxation techniques. It is not seen as a nice-to-have extra luxury, rather as a necessary part of the process of recovering from the trauma of cancer treatment. They also provide manual lymphatic drainage for every patient who has had axillary lymph node clearance, to reduce the risk of lymphoedema.

In Asian countries, integrative approaches are also used more widely. In China, Traditional Chinese Medicine (known as TCM) is part of the healthcare system. They have integrated hospitals where you can go to get your acupuncture and herbal medicine, alongside all the conventional treatment. If a person is treated in a Chinese hospital that doesn't offer TCM, it would be rare that they are not accessing it elsewhere. But it's not fully funded. And, while there are insurance plans, they don't necessarily cover everything. It is considered a reason why family relationships are so tight in China. If you get ill, your family will have to club together to pay for treatment.

All of which makes the NHS look pretty good in comparison (okay, maybe not compared with Germany). But, as we all know, the NHS is struggling right now. 'We're waiting for people to fall off the cliff before we treat them,' says Dr Fuller-Shavel. 'But that's ultimately more expensive. If we pick people up before they fall off the cliff, all of those metabolically unhealthy people stand a better chance. There are so many walking wounded who are considered healthy because they're able to go to work. But it costs people with their lives, in the long term. Sadly, nobody's looking at the long term.'

The complementary therapies quality gap

There is another issue at play here, which is that British people don't trust complementary therapies because they don't tend to come recommended by qualified medical professionals. And this isn't helped by the fact that the world of integrative oncology is not tightly regulated here. 'With the private healthcare system that they have in North America and Canada, they have a well-established system of complementary therapies,' explains Dr Fuller-Shavel. 'Naturopathic doctors actually go through formal training, just like medical doctors, which means a completely different level of education to naturopaths in the UK.' Naturopathy broadly describes any 'natural', ie. not medical, treatment. 'Australia is similar,' she continues. 'They have a rich naturopathic tradition, and the doctors have master's degrees or doctorates in naturopathic medicine. In the UK, they are not in any way medically educated.'

And part of the reason that lifestyle interventions are failing to break through into doctors' scope of awareness is that there is a distinct lack of people who are able to challenge the paradigm in a way that acknowledges the workforce and constraints in the public system. Unfortunately, it becomes a self-fulfilling prophecy because people don't trust naturopaths, and they don't get recognised training, so there are lots out there that are not very good.

So how do we make things better? 'What we hope to do at the BSIO is to create educational programmes,' she says. 'We already do monthly webinars about the most recent evidence across a broad range of topics for our members, who span doctors, nutritionists, naturopaths and yoga teachers. What we really want to do is establish a postgrad diploma or a master's in integrative cancer care. If we bring that in, people will learn about it properly and we can create a workforce across the three sectors to be able to deliver it properly. Because, if we don't educate, we don't have a workforce, and we can't deliver it. We've got to start with that.'

In her clinics, Dr Fuller-Shavel provides psychological, nutritional, lifestyle and complementary interventions that patients can use alongside their conventional cancer treatment. She tells me about one of her metastatic cancer patients, whose health improved so much under her care that he shocked his consultant. And improving quality of life for those with a terminal diagnosis is one of her passions.

'Look, I'm not sitting here promising miracles,' she says, 'but there is a need to focus on the human experience. It shouldn't just be: let's drug you up to the gills and then see what happens. Of course, medication is extremely important. But it's not health care, it's sick care.' And ideally we should be trying to prevent people getting sick in the first place.

Risk-reducing healthy habits

Reducing your risk of cancer is an area where an integrative approach can really help. Keeping your immune system in good working order is a good place to start. Here's why: most healthy people have cancer cells in their body. In fact, prostate cancer (the most common cancer in men) is often found to be present in men who have died of other causes: to the extent that you are 30 times more likely to die *with* prostate cancer than *of* it. And our immune system is designed to identify and destroy pre-cancerous cells, so anything we can do to support our body's resilience and immunity can reduce our risk. Innate self-healing mechanisms can sound pretty woo-woo initially but, if you look at the science, your body actually has an incredible capacity to heal and restore itself. Modern life – with its stress, pollution, processed convenience foods and devices that encourage us to be sedentary – does not provide the ideal conditions in which to thrive, so we have to make conscious choices.

Much of the advice may seem blindingly obvious. Your grandmother could have told you that it's important to slow down, eat your veg, drink enough water, get a good night's sleep and exercise. But the modern world tends to make you forget these basic tenets of good health, so it's helpful to develop strategies to ensure that you do them.

One strategy that's often talked about in terms of forming healthy habits is finding your 'why'. When you have a strong reason why you're implementing certain lifestyle changes, it's far easier to make them happen. And what better 'why' is there than avoiding the chemo ward? Meanwhile, many of these approaches can also help you cope with the psychological side of cancer treatment. The emotional stress of dealing with fatigue, skin rashes and chemo side effects such as hair loss and lack of libido should not be underestimated.

Cancer treatment is a rollercoaster. But, when you're in active treatment, you are at least on the rails. A doctor is in charge, and you can see where you are headed. People often find that they manage to stay strong throughout treatment. Then when treatment finishes, they come off the rails and suddenly feel anxious and abandoned, frighteningly out-of-control. So listen to your body and think about what you need and what to prioritise. If it's 'I can't stop crying', then psychological care should be at the top of your list. If you're feeling anxious and lethargic, then movement can help.

The joy of an integrated approach is that there is genuinely no downside. These approaches could help a lot and, at the very least, they won't do any harm. The only danger is if people start to believe that it's *all* down to their lifestyle choices. And whether or not the cancer comes back is due to whether they've meditated enough, or eaten enough broccoli. We can control many things in life, but we can't control everything. You could do every health intervention under the sun, optimising your physical and psychological wellbeing, and still get cancer. Although arguably it won't have been a waste of time, because you'll be in a better place to cope with treatment, physically and mentally.

My why

When I first started learning about this stuff, I felt a huge amount of pressure – that getting cancer was somehow my fault. I became obsessed with reading scientific studies about which lifestyle choices increase your risk of breast cancer, and picking out the behaviours of which I'd been 'guilty' at various points in my life. I drank too much in my 20s and 30s, I had a sedentary job and didn't exercise; I wasn't vigilant about additives in my food, I ate too much sugar when I was younger, I got too stressed at work, I had kids too late and didn't breastfeed for long enough . . . It took months for me to drag myself out of this pointless cycle of blame. With a family history of breast cancer, I was tested for the BRCA gene mutations that mean a higher risk, but it came back negative. This was good news; it means recurrence is less likely. But I was strangely disappointed, because I wanted a reason for my breast cancer. 'Whyyyyy has this happened?' I wailed to every doctor and expert I met. The answer was generally, 'it's just one of those things.'

Eventually, I realised that I have to accept it doesn't really matter why this has happened. I can't change the past. But what I can do is learn as much as possible about how to reduce my risk of recurrence in the future.

I really do want to live: I want to see my children become adults, and one day hold my grandchildren. Cancer truly clarifies what's important, and reaching those life milestones is a goal that feels absolutely vital to me right now.

If I'm going to practise what I preach and focus on the positives, then I can say that what I've been through has made me prioritise mine and my family's health. I'm utterly delighted that my experience and subsequent desire to live in a healthier way has rubbed off on my kids. Now my six-year-old daughter sings 'Vitamin Deeeeeee' as she twirls in the winter sunshine on a freezing February school run. And I chat with my eight-year-old son about the nutrients in food, while encouraging him to help me cook. He has never liked meat and announced aged five that he's a vegetarian, so I'm pleased that he now knows all about the best plant-based sources of protein.

Sugar, and the all-or-nothing fallacy

Certain lifestyle interventions can stress you out – attempting to stick to a restrictive diet can do more harm than good if it makes you feel deprived. Let's use the example of sugar. Most people know that, ideally, they should consume less refined sugar. Yes, our bodies need sugar, but the amount that we get from fruit, vegetables, carbohydrates and dairy is plenty. None of us needs to eat additional refined sugar, which can cause glucose spikes, increasing our risk of many conditions including cancer. But human beings are designed to crave sugar, and the emotional pull of a slice of birthday cake is hard to resist.

We have to learn to be easier on ourselves. With something like sugar or alcohol, you can end up in a vicious cycle of attempting to cut it out, falling off the wagon, and then feeling so demoralised that a binge seems like the only solution. That is no way to live. Instead, if you have a slice of cake, take the time to fully enjoy it. The stress of hating yourself for eating something is probably worse for you than the thing you're eating! And it can become a spiral of anxiety, leading to more binge eating, and on it goes. If you want to minimise your glucose spike, eat some protein or good fats before the cake, and then move your body afterwards. Then, focus on adding nutritious foods to your diet – meaning protein at every meal, and at least a couple of plant-based foods. The phrase 'plant-based' makes some people shudder at the thought of a joyless existence surviving on droopy salads, but plant-based means everything from fruit and vegetables to nuts and seeds, beans and chickpeas, herbs and spices, and oats and rice. It's honestly easier than you think to eat 30 different plant-based foods a week, which is what experts now recommend, rather than the 'five a day' advice on which I grew up. Focusing on what to include in your diet rather than what to exclude helps to crowd out less helpful food choices without feeling a bleak sense of deprivation.

Of course, if you're an all-or-nothing type who finds it easy to make a decision and stick with it, then cutting out alcohol, refined sugar and additives (anything on a food label that you can't pronounce) will instantly mean a healthier body. But most of us need to work at making healthy choices most of the time, and not beating ourselves up when we don't. I find it helpful to have a vague 80/20 guide in my mind, where I'm being healthy 80 per cent of the time, so it doesn't matter too much what happens in the other 20 per cent. Some weeks I'm very healthy, closer to 100 per cent of the time. Other weeks, I'm on holiday, or it's Christmas, so I let myself off the hook. Having rules can feel oppressive for some people. For me, it's a helpful guide. This is all about finding what works for *you*.

Having an open mind

If, at the end of this chapter, you're still not convinced, I'd advise you to try out a couple of the ideas mentioned earlier, and the more specific advice around nutrition, movement and mental health in the following chapters. When I was diagnosed with breast cancer, a nurse gave me a leaflet about complementary therapies on the NHS, but since we were in the third Covid lockdown none of them was actually available to me other than distance reiki. Now, I'm the kind of person who would be a bit cynical about the benefits of reiki in person, but *distance* reiki? It seemed so mad I wanted to see what it involved, so I signed up.

Each week while I was going through chemo, a man called Paul phoned me and we chatted about how I was feeling and any side effects I was experiencing. He would describe a visualisation or a breathing technique, and then we'd hang up and he would perform his reiki wherever he was, and I would supposedly feel the benefits, lying on my bed in East London. On paper, it sounds ridiculous. But the reality was that I had a set time each week when I could talk to a stranger about how I was feeling, and then lie in silence, focusing on my breathing or imagining the reiki doing me good. Do I believe that Paul's reiki vibes were pulsating across London and reaching me in Walthamstow? No, I don't. But did I find the experience intensely relaxing, and feel better afterwards? Yes! It was surely good for my nervous system and, in turn, my immune system. Something that started as a bit of a joke became an enjoyable stress-reliever and, in retrospect, a key part of my treatment. Of course, you have to give yourself over to it. If you lie there stewing on an argument or thinking about how pointless the whole endeavour is, then it's unlikely to do you much good.

It's like the placebo effect, it works if you believe it. When World War II doctor Henry Beecher ran out of morphine, he famously gave wounded soldiers saline injections, telling them it was pain relief, and was amazed when they started to feel better. It may sound like magical thinking, but it's just science: in response to feeling cared-for, patients' bodies produce their own drugs like dopamine and endorphins, which can reduce pain and make us feel calmer.

So take all the steps you need to feel like you're helping your body in the right direction. Give in to this idea of an integrated approach with a sense of realistic optimism, understanding that it's all about progress rather than perfection. Because being compassionate to yourself is the key. Behaviour change never comes from a place of shame or disappointment.

Anyone who has been through cancer treatment knows that one of the most difficult things about it is the lack of control you feel. Integrative care means clawing back some sense of agency, enabling supported resilience rather than learned helplessness. Sometimes that simply looks like a hard boundary of making time for yourself, which is otherwise hard to find. There are many, many reasons why people get cancer, but there's one thing I know for sure: it's not your fault. Be kind to yourself, and do everything you can to make your life a joyful, optimistic experience, in which your body feels nurtured. Lean into this new direction, even in a very small positive way, and you'll be surprised at where it can lead you.

Try something that you might not previously have thought of, whether small or big. It might be acupuncture, forest bathing or a gong bath - see what you make of it. And take some time to consider: What are the easiest lifestyle changes I can make right now? Make it easy and, even better, make it fun. Eat well, sleep well, move your body and find what makes *you* feel good.

TRY IT NOW

- Avoid glucose spikes by only having sugary foods after a balanced meal, and follow them with a walk, or any other form of movement, which will regulate your blood sugar.
- If you can't face cutting out alcohol entirely, then download an alcohol tracking app, as a step towards cutting back.
- Add more plant foods whenever you can, whether that's putting some seeds in your porridge, throwing a ball of frozen spinach into your pasta, or having fruit and veg snacks to hand for when you're peckish.
- Find simple ways to fit regular exercise into your day. Could you get up 20 minutes earlier and go for a walk before the rest of your household is awake?
- When arranging to meet a friend, see if they might be up for a walk or a yoga class, rather than going for a drink.
- Treat yourself as you would a child: make sure you get enough sleep, eat nourishing foods, move your body and find time to rest your mind and hang out with friends.

PART II:
TREATMENT

The following chapters are a practical guide to the different elements of cancer treatment, from chemotherapy and surgery, through radiotherapy and targeted treatments. Some women with breast cancer have surgery and radiotherapy, but not chemo. Some have chemo but don't need radiotherapy. And hormonal or endocrine treatments may be prescribed for those with hormone receptor positive cancers, but not for those with HER2 or triple negative breast cancer. These chapters are here to be dipped in and out of at the times when you most need them; turn to the one most relevant to you.

Surgery

For most of us, the operation during which the surgeon physically removes the tumour from your body will be the best possible action you can take against your cancer. Any kind of surgery can be scary, but particularly when it is life-saving surgery that alters the appearance of your body in such a hugely personal way. We will come to the psychological effects of breast cancer surgery shortly. But first, you may now be faced with some decisions to make about what kind of surgery to have.

Surgical options

Lumpectomy

Also known as breast-conserving surgery or wide local excision, this is when only a portion of the breast is removed along with the tumour. The surgeon will be looking for 'clear margins', which means a clear gap between the removed cancerous cells and remaining healthy tissue. There exist different views as to what constitutes an acceptable margin. It's usually said that surgeons aim for a clear margin of five millimetres, but many consider two millimetres acceptable, in certain circumstances. In some cases, a second surgery will be needed if the margins are not clear. Talk to your surgeon about what they are hoping to achieve with the surgery, and get them to explain clearly why they are recommending a lumpectomy rather than a mastectomy.

Mastectomy: unilateral or bilateral

When the entire breast tissue is removed, usually including the nipple. If the tumour is more than four centimetres across, or the disease is multifocal (more than one tumour in the breast), then a mastectomy will be strongly advised. Unilateral or bilateral refers to whether you are having one or both breasts removed. In most cases, a unilateral mastectomy will be sufficient to remove the tumour. But you might choose to have a bilateral mastectomy if you are at high risk of cancer in the other breast.

If you have a family history of breast or ovarian cancer (which is associated with increased risk), then you should be offered genetic testing to screen for mutations in the genes BRCA1 and BRCA2. More detailed screening can sometimes be available to check for TP53, PALB2, ATM and CHEK2, although these are less common. A genetic mutation will mean a recommended risk-reducing bilateral mastectomy, but you also can choose to have one if you are particularly anxious about recurrence, or even if you want a more symmetrical aesthetic result.

Surgeons are generally very honest about this, being clear with you if a mastectomy with reconstruction will actually look better afterwards. In my case, a mastectomy was the only option; since I had the most aggressive grade of breast cancer, the multifocal tumours represented a mass too large to remove by lumpectomy, and there was also lymph node involvement.

Axillary lymph node removal

This is the surgical removal of lymph nodes from your underarm. Your lymph nodes are the junctions at various points around the body that filter the flow of lymphatic fluid. These nodes under your arm are usually the first place that breast cancer cells reach, when spreading out of the breast. In my case, for example, the initial diagnostic ultrasound showed that at least two of the lymph nodes were swollen. I first had a fine needle biopsy of the area, which was inconclusive, so a further core biopsy was necessary (yes, a third biopsy, having already had one on each of the two breast tumours). This showed cancer was present in the lymph nodes. It can be difficult to tell exactly how many are affected without taking them all out. In some cases, the surgeon may remove one or two nodes, just to be sure that they are cancer-free. The number of axillary lymph nodes a person has under each arm can be anywhere between 10 and 40. I had full axillary lymph node clearance, where they are all removed. In my case, that meant 12 in total, of which three still showed evidence of cancer, even after five months of chemotherapy, so I was very relieved to have them all out. But full axillary lymph node clearance can lead to post-surgical complications, which we'll come to.

TISSUE MARKERS

You might have a small metal tissue marker, sometimes called a clip, inserted into your breast to mark the tumour. There are various types of marker, including ones made from titanium, and magnetic ones known as Magseed. You can't see or feel the marker once it's in place, and they can be used in different ways. I had two markers inserted immediately after my diagnosis, one in each tumour. This was so that, if my chemotherapy was so effective that the tumours shrank away to nothing, the surgeon would still be able to see exactly where they used to be. They are also sometimes inserted during lumpectomy surgery, so that the precise area can be targeted in any subsequent treatment, such as radiotherapy.

Reconstruction

Whether or not you want reconstruction, and what type of reconstruction, will depend on several factors. These include if it's a single or bilateral mastectomy, whether you're having radiotherapy after surgery, and your relationship with your breasts in the first place. Some people want to minimise the amount of surgery they need to have, and so choose to either go flat, or wear a prosthesis. I knew from the beginning that I wanted reconstruction. I was having a single mastectomy, and didn't want to look lopsided, but wanted a more permanent solution than a prosthesis. Each of the options have pros and cons, so it's a very personal choice.

Aesthetic flat closure

Choosing not to have reconstruction after a unilateral or bilateral mastectomy, also known as 'going flat', comes with the benefit of minimal surgical intervention. There is a whole online movement around 'going flat', with women getting incredible tattoos over the scars on their chest. If you think that might be for you, there is so much inspiration out there. Check out Flat Friends, a UK organisation dedicated to supporting women who have had mastectomy surgery without reconstruction.

Reconstruction with implant

This is when a implant is used to rebuild one or both breasts. If you're having a unilateral mastectomy, make sure you talk through every eventuality with your surgeon. Adjuvant treatments such as radiotherapy can impact breast implants, so it might be worth holding off until after that treatment has been completed, rather than having immediate reconstruction at the time of your mastectomy. Also have a discussion about how the reconstructed breast with an implant will look compared with your existing breast. There will be an opportunity for revision surgery a few months, or even years, down the line, to make your breasts more symmetrical. The benefit of a bilateral mastectomy is that both breasts should be pretty symmetrical immediately, but you will still be entitled to tweaks to improve the final appearance.

Reconstruction with expander

Some women choose to have what is called an 'expander', which is when saline is slowly pumped into a tissue expander in the breast over several months, before the permanent breast implant is placed. This is a good option if you want to have an implant but will be having radiotherapy after surgery. The saline injections encourage additional tissue growth to create a natural pocket for the implant. When it has reached the optimum size and shape, the tissue expander is removed and a permanent implant is inserted.

DIEP flap reconstruction

This is when one or both breasts are reconstructed using abdominal tissue, or sometimes tissue from elsewhere on your body. The acronym comes from the blood vessels, called deep inferior epigastric perforators, which are transferred to the chest, along with the skin and fat connected to them.

I chose to have immediate DIEP flap reconstruction for several reasons. I know women with implants who are happy with them and look great, but I personally felt uncomfortable with the idea of having a foreign body in my chest. This was particularly the case since I was only having one, and it would inevitably look different to my remaining breast. I'd also heard tales of implants needing to be replaced a decade down the line, which put me off. And the plastic surgeon advised me against an implant, since I was due to have radiotherapy shortly after surgery, and he said that can affect the appearance of breast implants.

DIEP flap reconstruction appealed to me because it was using my own tissue, rather than an artificial implant, and the breast would be softer and more natural. The surgeon explained that it would also age more naturally, and eventually 'droop' as I got older, like a real breast. Whereas an implant would stay unrealistically pert while my existing breast aged as normal.

While there are clearly many benefits to this type of reconstruction, it's important to be aware that it is major surgery, requiring a long period of recovery. The surgeon will make a large incision along your lower abdomen. If you've ever seen a C-section scar, it's in the same place but significantly longer, going from hip to hip. They will then remove the tissue before using microsurgery to attach the new 'breast' to small blood vessels in the chest wall. Since the abdominal skin is pulled tight, your tummy button will be replaced by a new incision. This part of the procedure was not mentioned to me before surgery, and I found it mind-bendingly weird to unexpectedly have lost my tummy button, on top of everything else. When you come round after surgery, you will be covered in a heated blanket to encourage blood flow in the new breast, and it will be checked regularly to ensure the blood is circulating well. You may feel very hot, claustrophobic and exhausted as, every time you manage to fall asleep, you'll be woken up for the next check-up. But being prepared for this is a step towards coping with it, as this intense part of the recovery is only for a few days. A DIEP flap also means a much longer operation than reconstruction with implants, and therefore a longer recovery.

Symmetrising surgery

After a lumpectomy or unilateral mastectomy, there should be a conversation about whether you can have symmetrising or revision surgery to achieve a better aesthetic result. This might take the form of a breast reduction or a breast lift on the other side (the cancer-free breast that has not been affected by surgery). In the case of a lumpectomy, your breast might only require a small amount of lipomodelling, where fat is taken from elsewhere on your body and injected into the breast, to fill the 'gap' left when the tumour was removed. You won't be able to have these conversations until at least three months after surgery, and many surgeons will say that it takes a year for everything to settle and for you to be able to see an accurate post-surgical result.

In the weeks after surgery, you may well struggle to come to terms with your new body. But do talk to your surgeon about anything that you're not happy with, because they are trained to understand. And the NHS is brilliant at acknowledging the psychological impact of breast surgery, so part of your treatment will include follow-up appointments with the plastic surgeon to determine if any further surgery is required to make your reconstruction look as natural as possible. In my case, this meant a minor bit of surgery to symmetrise the breasts.

At my first follow-up with the plastic surgeon, I pointed out that my reconstructed breast was bigger than my existing one, which made me feel wonky. My surgeon explained that it was intentional, as there is often 'shrinkage' after surgery, especially if you're going to have radiotherapy. Then, when there was still a difference in size 10 months after my mastectomy, he did a procedure that involved liposuction in the new breast, to make it closer to the same size as my other one. At the same time, I underwent another procedure – to build an artificial nipple, which involves making an incision and folding the skin up 'like origami'. The only step left for me is to have an areola tattooed on by a cosmetic tattooist, and then I might finally feel as though I have my right breast back.

Your decision

Please do take time to familiarise yourself with all of the options that are available, to make an informed decision. This is one area where I actually regret my own decision.

With a family history of both breast and ovarian cancer, I had the genetic test but it came back clear, so I agreed to a unilateral mastectomy. Then, in the week before my surgery, I met a woman who had chosen a bilateral mastectomy even though her genetic test results had also come back clear. When I asked why, she said her surgeon had explained that a diagnosis of grade three triple negative breast cancer, with the addition of family history, meant the risk of recurrence was high enough to warrant a bilateral mastectomy, even with a clear genetics result. The chances are, her surgeon explained, she may well have a genetic mutation that has not yet been identified. She was 40, like me, and had exactly the same diagnosis.

I quickly made an appointment to see my surgeon, who said that she could perform a bilateral mastectomy but that I did not have enough abdominal tissue for a double DIEP flap reconstruction. And, since they had already advised against implants before my adjuvant radiotherapy, it seemed my only option was to go flat for a few months, before reconstruction with implants could be done further down the line.

Thoroughly overwhelmed by this eleventh-hour turn of events, I asked my surgeon what she would do in my position. She said she would have the unilateral mastectomy, with the option to do the other breast, with reconstruction from tissue elsewhere on the body, at a later date. So I made a rushed decision, without checking with the plastic surgeon, and agreed to go ahead.

Three months after surgery, when I raised the idea of doing the other breast with the plastic surgeon, he said that it wouldn't be possible because I didn't have enough fat anywhere else on my body. My only reconstructive choice on the other side was now an implant, which would render pointless everything that I had just been through to achieve DIEP flap reconstruction on my right breast.

This is a situation where it would have made an enormous difference for me to have the breast surgeon and plastic surgeon in the same room at the same time. From what I have since learned about expanders and implants, I would have made a different choice. Learn from my mistakes, and do not rush into your decision.

WHAT TO ASK YOUR SURGEON

- How long will my surgery take?
- For how long will I be in hospital?
- What kind of margin are you expecting to achieve?
- Is there anything I should do pre-surgery to best aid my recovery?
- Which post-surgery bra do you recommend I buy, and does the hospital provide one?
- Will I have drains attached to me after surgery? How many?
- What is your advice for reducing swelling and scarring?
- What exercises should I be doing after surgery to regain mobility?
- If lymph nodes are being removed, what can I do to reduce my risk of lymphoedema?
- After a unilateral mastectomy, how long until we talk about whether I need/can have symmetrising surgery?
- Can I see examples of reconstructions that you have done?

Prehab

Most people know the concept of rehab, meaning the process of rehabilitation and recovery after surgery. But people are increasingly talking about 'prehab' – the steps you can take to prepare your body for surgery, and any other treatments you might be having.

Kat Tunnicliffe is an oncological physiotherapist at Perci Health. She would like to see cancer treatment start with 'front end' advice about both prehab and rehab, ideally at the point of diagnosis, to better prepare patients for what they're about to go through.

'It's where most cancer rehabilitation trials are being focused at the moment,' she says. 'I believe it can give our patients more of a sense of control, optimise their resilience and response to treatment, and ultimately reduce the risk of recurrence. Patients need to be informed as to where they can be signposted should they or their families need support, at any stage of their treatment journey – whether that be physical, nutritional, psychological, practical, financial, spiritual . . . the list is huge. If I had my way, there would be some kind of prehabilitation intervention before surgery, chemo, radiotherapy and hormone therapy, as they all have different impacts. The sooner that needs are identified, the better they can be managed, ideally with individualised care rather than a one-size-fits-all bombardment of leaflets.'

This prehabilitation would take the form of assessing postural issues, current fitness and activity levels, and managing any existing neck or shoulder problems, as breast cancer treatment will likely affect these areas, so they need to be treated sooner rather than later.

In terms of posture, this is something to pay close attention to after breast cancer surgery, as you might find that you subconsciously hunch over, as if to protect your scars. This can cause shortening of the muscles, which exacerbates postural dysfunction, and it becomes a vicious circle. This is particularly the case after DIEP flap reconstruction as the front of your body, from the lower abdominals upwards, will feel extremely tender and tight for several weeks, or even months, post-surgery.

Kat describes the point of diagnosis as a 'teachable moment' where every patient should be made aware of the most powerful take-home message: that exercise is clinically proven to improve treatment response and resilience as well as to reduce risk of recurrence in breast cancer. 'This puts our patients in a very strong position of contributing to their own recovery,' says Kat, 'which is hugely empowering. Particularly because the majority of its principles can be used across other long-term conditions such as obesity, diabetes and high blood pressure. So this ultimately improves the health and quality of life for people, enabling them to remain in work and utilise health services less.'

It would be win-win for the NHS and the economy in general. Someone should tell the prime minister. Kat says the thing she hears most often after post-surgical rehabilitation sessions is: 'Why did no one tell me this before?' That has got to change.

Also do your best to prepare yourself psychologically for surgery. Ask your surgeon for as many details about the day as they can provide, so you'll know what to expect. From having the cannula put in to administer the anaesthetic, to how soon you can expect to be able to get out of bed. I felt emotionally underprepared to be confined to a hospital bed for several days. Particularly since I was as good as attached to the bed, with two cannulas (including one in my foot), three drains, a catheter for urine, and mechanical cuffs strapped around my legs that intermittently filled with air to squeeze my calves and prevent deep vein thrombosis. And *then* the heated blanket on top of it all. Even writing this makes me feel sick and breathless at remembering how scared, claustrophobic and trapped I felt.

There is also a lot you can do pre-surgery to prepare your skin to be in the best position to heal well. Dryer skin leads to worse scarring, so keep the area well moisturised and ensure you're drinking lots of water and eating plenty of healthy fats, such as avocado, salmon, olive oil, nuts and seeds. It's particularly important to eat nutrient-rich whole foods if you're having surgery after chemotherapy, which can interfere with the absorption of nutrients through the gut lining.

Emotional stress is another factor that can affect our inflammatory status, which has repercussions in the skin. This is why conditions like eczema and psoriasis can be stress-related. So do practise whatever stress-management measures you can but don't feel under pressure to force yourself into some sort of artificially serene state at this point. I personally would not have taken kindly to somebody telling me to try and chill out in the run-up to my mastectomy!

WHAT TO PACK IN YOUR HOSPITAL BAG FOR SURGERY

These are ideas to help you practically plan, but different things are important to different people so think of your own needs. This list should inspire you, rather than being rigidly prescriptive. You might consider. . .

- An extra-long phone charger so you don't have to twist around to the plug socket.
- A water bottle with a straw, for ease of drinking. And the larger the better, so you don't have to fill it up as often.
- Facial wipes to stay fresh when confined to a hospital bed.
- An eye mask and ear plugs to help sleep during the day.
- Your own flannel and toiletries, to make that bed bath a nicer experience.
- Moisturiser and lip balm, as hospitals can be dehydrating environments.
- Healthy and comforting snacks to supplement the (often dreadful) hospital food.
- Headphones, or even headband earphones so you can sleep easily while listening to something lovely. Download podcasts, audiobooks and a soothing playlist.
- Talking of which, hospital Wi-Fi can be very hit and miss, so pre-load your phone or tablet with films or TV series to watch.

- A calming pillow spray will both counteract the medical smell, and help with sleep.
- If you're having DIEP flap reconstruction, I recommend a small fan to keep you cool under the sweaty heated blanket.

In terms of clothing...

- Button-up pyjamas or nightie, for ease of access to your chest.
- A dressing gown or long cardigan.
- Slippers or flip-flops that are easy to slide your feet into without having to bend over. Although you will be wearing those compression socks with grippy bottoms.
- The most important thing you need is a front-fastening compression bra. Those with a zip at the front, which can be easier than a fiddly hook and eye, are worth considering as it will be unfastened regularly for checks. You will wear it immediately after surgery, so ideally buy a dark colour, otherwise it will end up stained with blood or other surgery-related fluid. There are several specialist brands for post-surgery bras, including Amoena, AnaOno and Royce. If you're having a single mastectomy with no reconstruction, lots of these brands sell unilateral bras, which provide support for the remaining breast, and they also have options with a pocket for your prosthesis, if you're using one. They can be quite expensive but M&S also do a range, and even Primark launched post-surgery bras in 2022. And do ask your breast nurse about a bra, as some hospitals provide them.

Recovery

The amount of time it takes for you to feel active, or even mobile, again varies hugely depending on the type of surgery that you have had. After a lumpectomy, you may go home the next day and be doing normal activities within a couple of weeks. After a mastectomy with DIEP flap reconstruction, you're in hospital for a week, and physical recovery at home will take weeks, if not months. And there are other aspects that also play into recovery time, such as how long your surgery took.

'We know that anaesthetic times make a big difference to post-operative recovery,' explains oncoplastic breast surgeon Miss Georgette Oni. 'Having a one-hour anaesthetic is a huge difference compared to a five-hour anaesthetic. In my unit, if it's one side, we do DIEP flap reconstruction in four hours now. When you're doing both sides at the same time, it can take 10 hours, so you can see a big difference in patients that have had one side done versus two sides. After a 10-hour anaesthetic, it will take you days to get out of bed.'

Miss Oni's work is at the most technologically advanced end of the spectrum. In my case, even though it was only one side, surgery took 10 hours. When I woke up afterwards, I had a huge scar going from hip to hip across my lower abdomen. The skin across my tummy was stretched tight, and my tummy button had disappeared and been recreated by the surgeons. My right breast had been hollowed out, meaning much of the original skin remained. But there was now a circular patch of tummy skin sewn on to where my nipple used to be.

This was a really difficult part of the process for me. While I was grateful to the surgeons, I couldn't help feeling like a slab of meat that had been sliced up and put back together in the wrong way. It's not an exaggeration to say that it felt almost dehumanising. Having said that, my emotional response was exacerbated by the adverse reaction I had to the ketamine in the anaesthetic, which caused terrifying hallucinations all through my first night in hospital. And I wasn't allowed any visitors because of Covid restrictions, so was alone with my thoughts for five days.

Miss Oni says she has known people have hallucinations before, so I'm not a complete anomaly in that respect, and she says my difficulty in coping emotionally while in hospital is actually extremely common. 'What I have noticed with patients is, a couple of days after surgery, they get really, really upset and sad,' she explains. 'I call it the "day-two blues", and I think it's because they're actually getting over their anaesthetic, and seeing the reality of what's happened. It's very common for the patient to be teary as the gravitas of everything hits them.'

Talking to Miss Oni made me realise that my bad experience of surgery was actually quite preventable. Hopefully your surgery won't take as long as mine did, you will be more prepared for the emotional upheaval afterwards, and I certainly hope that you're not also dealing with a global pandemic preventing you from having any visitors.

But even with the best possible surgical scenario, I'm sure you'll still want to get out of hospital as soon as you can. Before you can be discharged, however, you have to be able to go to the bathroom all by yourself, meaning your catheter can be removed. You'll need lots of support at first, since moving around can be impeded by the fact that, initially, you may have several drains hanging out of your body. A drain is used to minimise swelling caused by fluid collecting in the wound cavity. It looks like a long plastic tube sticking out of your wound and attached to a bottle that slowly fills up with a grim-looking yellowy-pink fluid. You can actually buy specially designed bags to carry your drains, making it easier to walk around after surgery. I had three drains: one in my breast, one in my lymph node scar and one in my abdomen. The nurses told me that I needed to have all of my drains out before leaving hospital but, since then, I've heard of people going home with drains still attached and having them checked by a district nurse.

The other thing that needs to happen before you are allowed to leave hospital is, as the nurse put it, 'bowel movement'. Yes, the anaesthetic and painkillers can make you severely constipated, which is particularly unpleasant if you've had abdominal surgery. They will likely give you oral laxatives but if they don't work you can request a suppository, which they will pop up your bum and tends to do the trick! Make sure you drink lots of water too.

Depending on the type of surgery you have, rehabilitation can be a long process. Oncological physiotherapist Kat Tunnicliffe says it's really important that people manage their expectations around recovery. 'The side that has had surgery and/or radiotherapy will never structurally be the same as the unaffected side,' she says. 'It can be loaded, lengthened and used functionally as well as before. But we know from the evidence base that there are significant numbers of breast cancer patients left with persistent pain, joint and movement dysfunction, and a huge impact on quality of life.'

The answer to this is better wrap-around care, and more information for patients about how to prevent or improve post-surgical issues. So many people believe that if the doctor doesn't specifically tell them something, it's not important. And doctors rarely find time to tell you how vital it is to move your body, eat well and look after your mind. I wasn't given any post-surgical advice at all, other than a nurse mentioning in passing that I shouldn't lift anything too heavy. Others have reported being sent home with a highly sexist leaflet advising them not to do too much ironing, vacuuming and cooking. I've since realised the importance of movement after surgery, and feel quite let down that they didn't even give me the exercise lists that I understand are commonly distributed at other hospitals. Would it be that hard to create a standard list of practical dos and don'ts, which could be handed to *every* woman after breast surgery? Surely that's the least that should happen and, in Kat's professional opinion, support needs to go much further.

'As a bare minimum, physical, nutritional and psychological needs really do require closer attention,' says Kat. 'I know there are numerous patients out there who, through "survivor guilt", under-report their concerns. There is also that end-of-active-treatment cliff edge, where people feel abandoned with ongoing issues.'

The mind–body connection

Now, I know I said this section was about physical rather than psychological recovery but, according to Kat, they are intrinsically linked. 'The brain's perception of that upper quadrant is that it has had trauma after trauma after trauma,' she explains. 'If the system isn't flooded by "normal" fearless, painless movement, it will continue to be on high alert. This is why so much of physiotherapy is about restoring functional use. In the nicest possible way, it's an up-yours to the side effects and tissue reorganisation, by living the life you want to live. If your body is tight or weak, or if you're dealing with pain, instability or pelvic floor dysfunction, do not just put up with it as part and parcel of being cancer-free. Get help to live your best life possible. I hate the term "survivor"; I want my patients to thrive.'

Psychologically, there are also other ways in which our pain and weird sensations present themselves, or are expressed by the nervous system. This means factors such as low mood, disturbed sleep, lack of motivation to exercise, and intense fear of recurrence. Get help as soon as you can for any of these issues. Did you know that your GP can actually prescribe exercise on the NHS? I didn't, until recently, but they can hook you up with appropriate fitness classes in your local area, on prescription. Sadly, this happens quite rarely. I don't know whether many doctors don't realise they can do this, or if they think it doesn't work, but if you want to try it, just ask.

'The central nervous system is very sophisticated at telling us when something is not right or feels different,' says Kat, 'like that post-treatment feeling of your body just not being yours. Often, if you ignore it, it knocks on the door louder, amplifying what you're feeling or perceiving, in the expression of pain. Again, we know from strong evidence that remaining physically active is the best treatment for overcoming and reducing this. It's the best chance your central nervous system, and thus your body, has to feel as close to "normal" as it can.'

The physical issues that Kat sees most often after breast cancer surgery include:

- Pain and movement dysfunction due to tightness or weakness
- Sleep disturbances
- Swelling
- Cording
- Lymphoedema

If those last two words mean nothing to you, I can relate. I had no idea what either of them were until I started radiotherapy, two months after my mastectomy. It was only when I struggled to get my arms above my head on the radiotherapy table that the therapeutic radiographer pointed out I had very bad cording in my right arm, and told me that I should ask to be referred for physiotherapy. It was also a radiotherapy nurse who warned me about the risk of lymphoedema. About one in four women who have had full axillary lymph node clearance will develop one or both of these conditions, so they should have been explained to me before surgery. Hopefully they will be explained to you but, if not, read on and make sure you're informed as they *can* be avoided.

RECOVERY TAKEAWAYS

- Give yourself time, and proper lying-down rest. Your body has been through a lot.
- Keep on top of your pain relief medication, and understand the side effects of each. Co-codamol can exacerbate constipation, with which you might be struggling after the anaesthetic.
- If you weren't given any post-operative exercises on being discharged from hospital, give your breast care nurse a call and ask for them.

Cording

Cording is the say-what-you-see name for when a hard rope-like structure forms under the skin on the inner arm. No one seems to know exactly why it happens, although it's thought to be caused by inflammation and scarring of the tissue surrounding the vessels and nerves. 'Cords are commonly in the armpit,' says Kat, 'but can extend through the elbow into the hand, most commonly the thumb, and even along ribs and into the abdomen.' It can be painful, and the tightness can seriously reduce your range of movement, which is why I initially struggled to get my arms above my head on that radiotherapy table.

When I first noticed the cording a few weeks after surgery, I was terrified to touch it because I thought it was some kind of tendon or ligament that I might accidentally damage. It was reassuring when the physiotherapist explained that it was actually hard tissue, and firm massage would improve it. Having said that, I still didn't like to touch it, and made Jonathan massage it firmly while I did a hard stare in the other direction.

Kat acknowledges that the massage can be uncomfortable, but says it shouldn't hurt too much, and definitely won't cause lasting damage. 'It's important to know that a popping sound or sensation can occur when the cords are released, but this is not causing any damage, and it doesn't always happen,' she explains. 'Some surgeons evoke so much fear in our patients by telling them to "go see the physio to get your cords snapped". Either way, the earlier the cording is treated, the better the outcome. It appears most commonly in the healing phase, although some can get it months or even years later. If that's the case, I would always get it checked for anything else going on in the lymphatics.'

CORDING TAKEAWAYS

- Get those exercises and do them!
- If you don't feel your recovery is going as it should, ask to be referred to a physiotherapist (some hospitals arrange a physio as standard but, if not, just ask).

Lymphoedema

Oedema is a condition where a build-up of fluid in the body causes uncomfortable swelling. Lymphoedema, therefore, is when the fluid involved in this process is lymph fluid. Don't worry if this is completely new to you. Pre-cancer, the only context in which I had heard of the lymphatic system was seeing 'lymphatic drainage' as a massage option on a spa treatment list.

Usually, when bacteria enters the lymphatic system as an infection, it is transported to the lymph nodes, where it is destroyed. This is why lymph nodes are important; they're like a filter for your lymphatic system. 'Think of the lymphatic system like the M25,' says Kat Tunnicliffe. 'The lymph fluid is the traffic, lymph vessels are the lanes, and the nodes are the junctions. If a junction is removed, the road is closed. Thus alternative routes need to be found to minimise fluid collecting in the arm or hand.'

If that process doesn't happen, then it can cause pain and swelling, which can become quite severe. When the actress Kathy Bates had breast cancer surgery, she described lymphoedema as 'psychologically so damaging; it was almost worse than having cancer.'[2] This is many people's experience, so it's really worth being prepared.

The good news is that your body is resilient and adaptable. Over time, your lymphatic system will adjust, and other lymph nodes will compensate for the missing ones. If you have had only a few lymph nodes removed, not full clearance, then you are very unlikely to have any serious issues. Even if you have had full clearance, you have more lymph nodes in your neck, chest and groin that will start to compensate for your missing ones.

The less-good news is that lymphoedema is incurable so, once you have a diagnosis, it's something you have to manage for life, rather than being able to successfully rectify it for ever. If you already have a lymphoedema diagnosis, don't panic. I do too, and there is plenty that you can do to support your lymphatic system and keep symptoms at bay.

Kat says that one of the best exercises for moving that fluid around is co-contraction, when muscles act in opposite directions of the same joint. Pilates is great for this. And you should be given a list of simple arm exercises to do after your surgery. If you are not given these, ask again, as they're really important for reducing your risk of post-surgical complications and improving your range of movement. There's a lot of fear around exercising after this type of surgery, and the only advice I was given was to rest, and not lift anything too heavy. This frustrates physiotherapists like Kat immensely, and she tells me she is very keen to quash the myths around movement after breast cancer surgery.

'Out-of-date advice about avoiding use of the affected arm encourages fear and results in inactivity,' she says. 'Any activity is better than nothing. We now know that we can lift weights, although it is important to be done in a paced and graduated way, as "eager beavers" who push too hard, too quickly can result in inadequate lymphatic drainage before the system has recovered.'

Brilliantly, I was guilty of both inactivity and overdoing it. I was initially fearful of using my right arm, and ended up with quite severe cording. Then, when I realised how important movement is to recovery, I threw myself into yoga too soon. All those planks and downward dogs resulted in (thankfully quite mild) lymphoedema in my right hand and wrist. I now know that yoga is fine, but putting your entire body weight on the affected wrist too soon is not. What 'too soon' actually means will be different for everyone. I was six months post-surgery, so thought it would be fine. Nevertheless I certainly powered through my planks and downward dogs, despite discomfort and swelling in my right hand. Learn from my mistakes, and listen to your body. Now, I still do planks but on my elbows rather than my wrists, and any decent yoga teacher should be able to adapt the exercises if you tell them what kind of surgery you've had.

The other thing is not to panic when you hear a doctor say that lymphoedema is 'incurable'. I was so scared when I first heard this, and thought I would permanently have one swollen hand and wrist, which would always look strange compared to my other side. But what I learned is that lymphoedema is 'incurable' in a similar way to something like a cold sore. You'll always have to be aware of it as something that can flare up, often when you're rundown or haven't been taking care of yourself. But that doesn't mean it's always visible. I manage it by wearing a compression glove during exercise, and ensuring I drink enough water, get enough sleep and avoid alcohol and processed foods. I've also found reflexology to be hugely effective in keeping it under control. If I let those things slide (over

Christmas, for example), then I will wake up with sausage fingers – which is a good reminder and incentive to prioritise my health a bit more!

'You can also stimulate the skin directly, such as with lymphatic massage, brushing and swimming or other exercise in water,' says Kat. 'The incidence of lymphoedema increases in those that are less active and overweight, because of too much load squashing the vessels so that adequate flow can't be reached. Your heart and diaphragm are important "pumpers" so need to be working effectively. I do a lot of work on posture and workspace ergonomics to reduce the "crumpling" effect on the diaphragm.'

While lymphatic massage is great, you might find that some spas and salons don't like to do it if you've had full axillary lymph node clearance, although there's no real reason for this other than inexperience. There are beauty and massage therapists that are trained in the specific challenges facing cancer patients, and you can find one through an organisation called Wellness for Cancer. Either way, always make sure the therapist knows that you've had this type of surgery so they are not sweeping the lymph towards an area with no lymph nodes.

Nurses and phlebotomists will often ask if you've had lymph nodes removed before doing a blood test or taking your blood pressure, and then avoid the affected arm. This is because of the tightness of the tourniquet or arm cuff pressing down on the vessels, which can increase your risk of lymphoedema.

You should also avoid anything that breaks the skin on the affected arm, such as tattoos or piercings and even acupuncture. I was advised not to have manicures, but have since learned it's actually fine if you trust the salon to keep everything sterile, and ask them not to cut your cuticles. Taking good care of your skin with regular moisturising and avoiding sunburn is also important for many reasons, but specifically in this case to prevent infection.

If you're interested in going deep with lymphatic knowledge, there is a great book by Lisa Levitt Gainsley called *The Book of Lymph: Self-Care Practices to Enhance Immunity, Health and Beauty*. It's a really brilliant guide to one of the body's main functions, one we barely think about, until we have to.

LYMPHOEDEMA TAKEAWAYS

- Regular exercise is important to keep your lymph flowing, but don't put your body weight on your wrists (as in a plank or push-ups).
- If you feel swelling in your hand, wrist or arm, ask your breast nurse for a compression glove or sleeve, which prevents fluid build-up.
- Reduce your risk of infection in that arm by avoiding breaking the skin where possible. Wear sun block and insect repellent when needed.
- Light self-massage or body brushing can be good for lymph flow, but ensure you are not brushing fluid towards the area where the nodes were removed. Cancer Rehab PT is a YouTube account with lots of videos on how to do it properly.
- I found reflexology really effective for managing lymphoedema, but make sure your reflexologist is trained in specific lymphatic techniques.

Scarring

Scarring is part of the body's natural healing process, where collagen is produced to form new fibres around a wound and heal the skin. But it can take two years for scars to flatten and fade. And, when your scars are associated with a traumatic event like cancer treatment, they can be a painful daily reminder.

It took a long time for me to be able to look at my scars, let alone touch them. Emma Holly is a scar therapist and founder of Restore Therapy Scar Clinic. She tells me that my distraught reaction on waking up to a mutilated body is very common. Even though you rationally know why it has happened, it's still a huge physical and emotional trauma. 'There's a big psychological element around people not liking to touch their scars,' she says. 'It's understandable because they're a constant reminder of the cancer, and there's a whole lot of anxiety and stress around that.'

The only real answer to that is time. And, while your emotional scars are healing, you will probably also want to do all that you can to reduce your physical ones too. Scar creams, gels and silicone strips can be effective, as well as massaging the area. You can start using these as soon as the scars have healed over, so there is no more bleeding or scabbing. How long this takes will vary from person to person, and surgery to surgery, but it's generally around three weeks.

Depending on what kind of surgery you've had, scarring might be quite extensive, so it's a good idea to bite the bullet and touch your scars as soon as you can face it. 'Scar creams do work, it's not just all about advertising,' says Emma. 'In early healing, when it's really fragile and thin, the body puts down scar tissue because the usual barrier of the skin is not there. A good quality scar product helps the body by providing a temporary barrier, minimising the risk of a scar becoming hypertrophic, which means it's red and raised, or keloid, meaning it grows really big.' In this instance, silicone scar strips can be a big help, not least because you can simply lay them over the scar without having to touch it too much. But scar creams containing silicone are also very effective.

'Another thing that causes an inferior cosmetic result is if there's a lot of tension on the scar,' continues Emma. 'For example, if a woman has large breasts and undergoes a lumpectomy, the weight of the breast can be dragging on the scar. I'd recommend wearing a good compressive bra until it's well healed, because that is going to make a much wider scar.'

Mechanomodulation is the unnecessarily convoluted word used to describe how massage will improve the appearance of your scars by stimulating healthy cells. The good news is, if you're cautious about touching your scars, you don't have to press hard. In fact, Emma explains, it's often better if you don't. 'Self scar massage should be gentle in my opinion. Some people will recommend very vigorous massage but more recent research leans towards too much pressure causing more inflammation and making scar tissue worse. Actually, a lot of scar tissue is superficial, so you shouldn't have to press that hard to generate change.'

As my plastic surgeon told me, the goal of reconstruction used to be that your breasts would look fine in clothes. Nowadays, however, the aim is that someone could see you topless and not know you've had a mastectomy – and with modern techniques, that can be a reality. While I think it's important to manage expectations around scarring and post-surgical complications, I also want you to feel optimistic and hopeful about the whole process, because it can lead to amazing results.

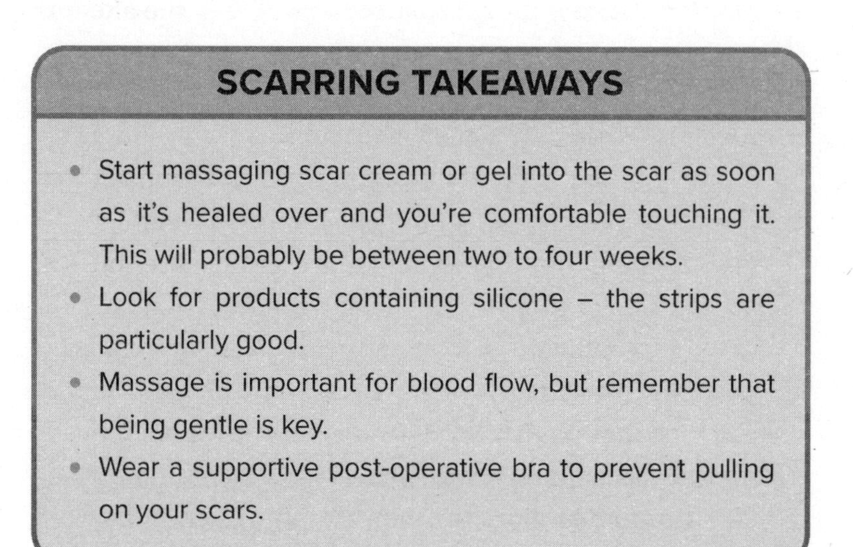

SCARRING TAKEAWAYS

- Start massaging scar cream or gel into the scar as soon as it's healed over and you're comfortable touching it. This will probably be between two to four weeks.
- Look for products containing silicone – the strips are particularly good.
- Massage is important for blood flow, but remember that being gentle is key.
- Wear a supportive post-operative bra to prevent pulling on your scars.

Psychological recovery

From puberty, if not before, girls are taught by society that breasts are intrinsically linked to womanhood and femininity. Our breasts are sexualised, but also associated with motherhood and that caring, nurturing role. Everywhere you look, from advertisements to Instagram to *Love Island*, the idea portrayed is that women's bodies are synonymous with women's value to society, and breasts play a key role in that.

If you're premenopausal, and would like to have children after cancer treatment, then you might have to come to terms with the idea that breastfeeding might not be possible. If you're not in a relationship and would like to be, then there will likely be fear of sexual rejection because of your new post-surgery body.

Even if you are able to have breast-conserving surgery, known as a lumpectomy or wide local excision, rather than a full mastectomy, it may still change the shape of the affected breast. And if you do have a single or bilateral mastectomy, whether you opt for reconstruction with implants or DIEP flap, or no reconstruction at all, there will be scarring.

It's really important to acknowledge these fears and address them, as it can be easy to assume you should feel nothing but gratitude to be having life-saving surgery. Of course, human beings are capable of feeling more than one thing at a time. So you can feel simultaneously grateful and relieved about the surgery that will remove the cancer, while also feeling scared and anxious about how your new body will look and feel, and what it will mean for your future relationships – not least your own relationship with your body and how that impacts your confidence. If you feel ready, try and reframe your anxiety around surgery to a sense of excitement. After all, this is the day on which you are taking the biggest step towards being cancer-free.

Learning to love, or at least feel comfortable in, your post-surgery body will take time. Give yourself that time to feel what you need to, whether that's sadness, anger or grief for your old body. Don't sweep your feelings under the carpet and put on a brave face. But also think clearly and rationally: you can't yet predict the aesthetic outcome as everything fluctuates so much in the year after surgery. Once your scars have healed, your surgeon will be able to talk you through the next steps, if required. Understand that it takes time. Be kind to yourself, seek professional psychological support if you feel it will help (your breast nurse can refer you for that) and understand that everything you're feeling is a one-hundred-percent normal and reasonable reaction to what you're going through.

Chemotherapy

When people think of cancer treatment, the first thing that comes to mind is chemo. And for good reason. If chemo is part of your treatment plan, it will likely be the most gruelling and emotionally draining element of the whole process. Having said that, it doesn't mean that you will become the fragile, bald-headed figure that has become emblematic of cancer treatment.

First of all, the facts. Chemotherapy is a treatment involving drugs - either used alone or in combination with others - to kill cancer cells. They do this by identifying fast-multiplying cells and destroying them. This makes them very effective in attacking tumours, but any part of your body that grows or regenerates also involves multiplying cells, which is why chemo can have a devastating impact on your hair, your nails and other parts of your body; a subject we'll cover shortly.

Despite being widely thought of as the main element of treatment, many breast cancer patients actually don't require chemo, and others are given the information and the chance to weigh up the statistics against the experience of going through chemo, to make their own decision.

In my case, it was a no-brainer. I was told that 16 rounds of chemo over five months was necessary to shrink the tumours in my right breast before surgery, so I never looked at percentages.

I didn't ask for a second opinion because I could see the logic of shrinking the tumours before surgery, particularly since there were also cancer cells in the lymph nodes. But, if yours is a more borderline case, a second opinion is always an option. The NHS can refer you for one, you don't have to pay privately for it (although, of course, you can if you want to). I later learned through the NHS Predict breast cancer tool that mastectomy surgery reduced my chance of death over the next five years by 42 per cent, with chemotherapy adding another 18 per cent benefit, so it was definitely worth it. But I know others for whom surgery was 75 per cent of the survival benefit, with chemotherapy representing less than a further 5 per cent.

Go through all of your options with your surgeon and oncologist because, in my case, chemo was very necessary, but in yours it might not be.

The jargon

The purpose of neoadjuvant chemotherapy (i.e. before surgery) is to shrink the tumour before removing it. The purpose of adjuvant chemotherapy (after surgery) is to blitz any stray cancer cells that might be remaining in the body after surgery. If you have chemo, the decision about whether to have it before or after surgery will depend on many factors, including the size, type and grade of your tumour.

As you know by now, there are many variables between different types of breast cancer, so the drugs you are prescribed may be different to the person with breast cancer in the chemo chair next to you. I'm not going to go into every single chemo drug here, because that would make for extremely dull reading, and they are all listed on the Cancer Research UK website, where you can find all the facts about your specific drug. This is useful and reassuring for those nights when you start to wonder if the side effects you're experiencing are normal, or if you ought to be more worried, or even contact someone about it. Of course, that information is also all in the leaflet the oncologist gives you when you sign the consent form, but who knows where *that* leaflet is when you're having a 2 a.m. wobble.

What I can do is tell you about my experience, and talk you through the side effects, which are broadly similar across all chemotherapy drugs for breast cancer.

First, I had four fortnightly rounds of AC chemo, which is a combination of doxorubicin and cyclophosphamide. Then I had 12 weekly cycles of paclitaxel and carboplatin, known as Taxol/Carbo for short.

AC chemo is often known as 'the red devil' due to its colour, which disconcertingly re-emerges as bright red urine. Infusions are usually two or three weeks apart, to allow the body to recover, and your medical team will keep a close eye on your heart and liver function, as these can be affected by treatment. The nausea and hair loss were most intense during those first eight weeks on AC chemo. The Taxol/Carbo, which is a common combination used to treat other cancers including lung, ovarian and cervical, I found easier to cope with in terms of side effects. In total, my neoadjuvant chemotherapy took 20 weeks.

I was also prescribed adjuvant chemotherapy after surgery. This was because I did not have a complete response to chemo

– meaning the pathology result of surgery showed there was still some cancer in the breast and lymph nodes.

I was prescribed capecitabine, which is taken in pill form and has fewer brutal side effects than the intravenous chemo I'd had previously. Importantly (for me anyway), hair loss was not one of them, so I managed to hold on to the fluffy regrowth that I had at that point.

PICC line

With intravenous chemotherapy, your treatment will be regularly administered over a period of weeks or months. This means that you may be fitted with a PICC line or a port, for ease of connecting you up to the infusion. This is good news for those of us with difficult veins, particularly if you've had distressing experiences in the past with medical professionals struggling to take blood or get a cannula into your arm.

A PICC line is a tube inserted through the arm (above the elbow) and threaded through a vein that goes up into your chest and down into one of the large arteries. You may also be offered a central line, which is a similar thing, but the tube goes under the skin on your chest.

This is what I had and, while it sounds grim, it's actually painless to have inserted. It stayed there throughout my five months of chemo, which was brilliant in terms of making chemotherapy sessions a needle-free experience, but it was inconvenient in other ways.

A PICC line is held in place by a device called a stat lock, and is usually neatly tucked away under a dressing, but it does mean you have a loose bit of tubing hanging out of your arm at all times and you can't help being aware of it. You have to keep it dry, and every week it must be flushed to prevent infection and have the dressing changed. You will have to stow away any tight-sleeved knits, as looser sweatshirts and hoodies will be more comfortable. I bought a soft, oversized hoodie with a zip, for ease of access to my arm during chemo, which I basically lived in throughout treatment.

If you have any pets or small children, you'll be advised to keep them away from your arm. And, considering my kids were only six and three at the time, I have to give them credit for remembering they could no longer grab me where the PICC line emerged – most of the time, anyway.

One of my initial concerns with the PICC line was that I worried I wouldn't be able to have a bath. I know, that sounds like a small thing, but a bath had become one of my small joys during lockdown. I wasn't about to give that up now that I needed as many anxiety-busters as I could find. Happily, I discovered a waterproof PICC line cover that would allow me to keep that part of my arm dry in the bath and shower. The one I bought was from a brand called Limbo, but there are lots of them out there.

Overall, I'm glad I had a PICC line, but I sure was happy the day I had it taken out.

Port

A port, otherwise known as a portacath or subcutaneous port, is a soft plastic tube that is connected to a large vein above your heart. It is accessed by a disc-shaped opening just under the skin on your chest, or sometimes on your inner arm. It requires a small surgical procedure to put it in, which is usually done under local anaesthetic, and you can go straight home afterwards. You'll be able to see and feel a small bump under your skin when it's in place. During chemo, the skin over the port will be numbed with anaesthetic cream, and the nurse will then push a special needle, called a Huber needle, through the skin and into the port. It might feel a bit weird but shouldn't be painful. The benefit of a port compared to a PICC line is that it doesn't interfere with your daily activities in the same way. You don't need to wear a dressing over it, and can have a shower or bath without having to cover it up. You can even go swimming – although this does carry a small risk of infection. It's therefore a better option for somebody having longer-term treatment. There should be a certain amount of choice, depending on your general health and the length of your treatment programme, so have a chat with your oncologist about the best option for you.

Steroids

Steroids are prescribed as tablets during chemotherapy, and generally have two functions. Alongside chemo drugs such as paclitaxel, they're given to reduce the risk of an allergic reaction. So, if you've had that drug two or three times, then you should be able to decrease the amount of steroids because the risk of allergic reaction goes down. The more common use for steroids is that they can be a powerful anti-nausea drug. You might quite reasonably think, then why am I taking these other anti-nausea drugs? But many of them actually work better when combined with steroids and so are more necessary than they may seem.

I didn't actually know any of the above until I researched it for this book. No oncologist ever explained to me why steroids had been prescribed; they were simply part of the battery of drugs that I was handed and obediently took during those first months after my diagnosis.

However, many people (me included) struggle with the side effects of steroids, which can include insomnia, mood changes such as anxiety and irritability, increased appetite and weight gain, and fluid retention leading to that dreaded puffy 'chemo face'. That doesn't seem so bad when written down but, believe me, it can be emotionally destabilising, particularly when combined with hair loss, including eyebrows and eyelashes.

I actually reduced my dose of steroids over time, because I struggled with the side effects and, since no one had explained what they were for, I didn't see the point of them. But I did so without telling my oncologist because I was worried that they would instruct me to keep taking them anyway. Looking back, this was madness. My oncologist would absolutely have explained everything fully, had I asked her to, and it's so important to have this open dialogue.

You will probably be advised to take them initially but, if you want to, you can have a conversation with your oncologist about reducing your dose once you're in the swing of treatment. It is not advisable to stop taking steroids abruptly, as this can lead to side effects including serious nausea, breathlessness and dizziness.

WHAT TO PACK FOR CHEMO INFUSION DAYS

- Your Cancer Treatment Record. This is the blue book given to you when you start chemo, in which the nurses will record your treatment every time you go.
- A large bottle of water, as hydration is key. Just remember to use the bathroom before your infusion begins, as it's a bit tricky once you're hooked up, especially if you're using the cold cap.
- Headphones, plus something to watch, read or listen to. Make sure you download what you need in advance, as hospital Wi-Fi is rarely fast and reliable.
- A snack. Some people choose to fast during chemo, and you'll know whether that's right for you, or if being hungry will make you more uncomfortable. In my experience, the food available on the ward is not the healthiest or the most appetising, so I always had an almond butter sandwich and an apple in my bag.
- A large scarf, hot water bottle or a heated pad if you're using the cold cap.
- Make sure you're wearing something comfortable, and ideally front-fastening, for easy access to your PICC line or port, if you have one.

Neutrophils

Before each round of chemo, you will have a blood test to check your neutrophil levels. It will also check on your platelets, which is to do with your blood clotting effectively, and your haemoglobin, or red blood cell count, which is your iron levels.

Your white blood cells, or neutrophils, are important because they help your body fight infection and heal injuries. Sadly, chemotherapy tends to attack them, which is why you will likely find that during treatment you'll pick up every cold that's going around and, if you cut yourself, it will take longer than usual to heal. For chemotherapy, they generally look for a neutrophil count of greater than 1 or 1.5. However, this can vary. For example, one chemotherapy nurse told me that they would go ahead with my treatment even if my neutrophil count was on the borderline because I was an otherwise healthy 40-year-old. With someone much older or generally more frail, they would be more careful, so don't get too hung up on the numbers.

Platelets and haemoglobin are also affected by chemotherapy. You may find that you suddenly start having nosebleeds, or realise you are covered in unexplained bruises, which can be a result of a low level of platelets in the blood. Low haemoglobin, or anaemia, can have significant implications in terms of fatigue. But the main purpose of the pre-chemo blood test is to check on the neutrophils because they need to be at a certain level for your body to tolerate the infusion. Looking after yourself in general, such as eating well, exercising and getting enough sleep, will also help your body produce more neutrophils.

Regular blood tests are an important part of chemotherapy, so one of the great things about having a PICC line or a port is that they can take blood painlessly through that. However, this does require you to be able to get to the chemo ward on blood test days, since normal phlebotomy clinics in your local surgery or hospital may not have the equipment or training to take blood in that way. Lots of people will find their chemo ward is some distance away from their home, so they will have to weigh up how far they are prepared to travel to avoid a standard needle-in-the-arm blood test.

BLOOD TESTS

There are people for whom a blood test is a walk in the park: a brief sharp prick with a needle, and then home. Others find them a stressful ordeal of many jabs in different places as the nurse struggles to find a vein that will produce blood. Unfortunately, I am in the latter group. My veins are apparently tiny and hard to find, and I've had nurses work themselves up into a frenzy as they try and fail to get a vein – in both of my arms, the back of my hand, my wrist and once, horrifically, in my foot. Over the years, I have picked up some tips to make the process easier.

- Go to a blood clinic where you'll see a phlebotomist who takes blood all day, every day. They really know what they're doing. Doctors do it so rarely that, frankly, it's often a shambles.
- Drink lots of water ahead of the test, as that helps with blood flow.

- Move your body as much as possible. Walk to the clinic, pace around the waiting room, stretch your arms and pump your fists, again to help with blood flow.
- Keep your body warm, so if it's a cold day do wrap up well.
- Make your phlebotomist relaxed and happy. If they casually ask whether people normally have any trouble with your veins, I have learned to smile and say, 'No, it's usually fine!' Otherwise they are stressed from the offset, which doesn't help anyone. I also like to throw them a compliment at the end: 'You're so good at that, it was basically painless!' I see this as paying it forward to the next person in the chair.
- Try and relax. I know this is easier said than done but, for thousands of years before modern life, a stressful situation almost always meant a physical threat. Because of that, your body's stress response is preparing for physical assault. Your veins do literally shrink away from the surface of your skin, and your blood can actually become stickier. It's the body trying to protect itself so, if you're injured, you will lose less blood. Clearly, though, this biological response doesn't help in a blood-test situation.
- Practise taking some deep breaths and, as you do, breathe in calm and breathe out anxiety. You might feel silly initially but, to be honest, I increasingly care less and less about what other people think. So, if you ever see me waiting for a blood test, I'm the one pacing around, pumping my fists between sips of water and breathing out my anxiety.

- If you have a PICC line or a port, and you'd prefer to have blood taken painlessly through that, then you have to go to the chemo ward. They prefer you to do this a couple of days before treatment, but many hospitals will allow you to come in early and do your bloods first thing. I personally preferred to do it all in one day, rather than have a separate trip to the blood clinic a couple of days earlier, when my neutrophils were often not high enough so they'd end up repeating it on the chemo ward anyway. You will have a wait, usually at least two hours, before you can have treatment. But my chemo ward provided buzzers so that they could buzz me when it was ready, meaning that I could go and wait in the Maggie's centre on the hospital grounds. This whole thing does make for a longer day at the hospital, but I used to take my laptop and use that time in Maggie's quite productively.

How to increase your neutrophil count

Your neutrophils form a key part of your immune defences, so think about the advice that is usually thrown around when it comes to protecting yourself against any kind of illness:

- Eat plenty of fruit and vegetables
- Drink lots of water
- Get regular quality sleep
- Move your body more often
- Find ways to relax, and manage emotional stress
- Drink less alcohol

As well as all of this, and depending on the type of chemo you're having, you may also be prescribed Filgrastim, which helps the bone marrow produce more neutrophils.

Filgrastim comes in a set of syringes that must be kept in the fridge, and you have to inject yourself (or get someone else to do it) every evening for a few days after your chemotherapy session. In my case, I had Filgrastim injections for four days after each AC chemo, but I didn't need them during the Taxol/Carbo. Whether you are prescribed it, and how much, will depend on many factors including your height and weight and general health. They say that a common side effect of Filgrastim is bone pain, but I didn't experience that. I'm not a fan of needles, and I don't think Jonathan loved injecting me in the tummy, but other than that this was actually one of the easier aspects of the whole process.

WHAT TO ASK YOUR MEDICAL ONCOLOGIST

- What will be the hormonal effects of my treatment?
- Will I have a PICC line or a port, and do I have a choice?
- What is your advice for things I can do at home to support myself through treatment?
- Can I talk to you about reducing the dose of my steroids or anti-sickness pills if I'm struggling with side effects of those during treatment?

- If I drive to chemo, are there discounted parking rates for chemo patients? (There is often discounted local parking, and Londoners can have the Congestion Charge reimbursed.)

Side effects

As we've already discovered, most chemo drugs work in a similar way: by identifying and destroying fast-multiplying cells. This means they attack your skin, your nails, your womb, the inside of your mouth, your stomach lining and, most noticeably (to other people anyway), your hair. While those might be the most painful and visible ones, the drugs affect every cell in your body to some extent, which can lead to many varied side effects.

You might feel pretty helpless initially, but there is actually a lot that you can do to reduce the severity of the side effects, and there is a huge amount that I wish I'd known before I started chemo. It's frustrating to think back and realise that so many of things that helped me were picked up randomly along the way, in the form of advice from other women that had been through it, on online forums or social media. In an ideal world, there would be more officially prescribed lifestyle advice, because there are plenty of (often quite small) things that you can do to improve how your body tolerates treatment. The important thing to remember is that you don't have to suffer any side effects in silence. If your lifestyle isn't helping, there will be a drug that can. Use every tool available to you at this point.

Tiredness and fatigue

This can become quite extreme, as every cell in your body strugglestocopewiththeonslaughtofchemo.It'snotahungover-but-coping tiredness: it's a bone-deep, can't-get-out-of-bed exhaustion. Now is the time to take care of yourself, physically and mentally, as you probably have never done before. For most of us, the responsibilities and demands of modern life mean that we rarely carve out time for ourselves, so cancer treatment can be something of a self-care crash course. It means early nights. It means saying no to things you don't want to do – and some things that you do. It means letting go of your to-do list and allowing yourself to watch a movie or read a book, or just have a nap, without feeling like you ought to be doing something else. It means running a bath instead of attending to life admin. And allowing others to pick up the slack.

I am fully aware that all of this is much easier said than done – believe me, I know it's hard. And I'm aware that it's actually a rarity and a privilege to feel cared for. There is such an emphasis on self-care these days, which can be great, but don't let it be at the expense of letting other people take care of you. I refer you again to the 'How can I help?' list on *page 45–46*. Show that to people or find other ways to make friends and family explicitly aware that a chemo patient might not have the energy to ask for help, but any practical help is gratefully received at this time.

Acknowledging how important it is that you give your body a chance to regroup after each cycle of chemotherapy is the first step towards actually doing it. Exercise has been proven to reduce the effects of fatigue and so, even though it might be the last thing you feel like doing, it's worth finding time to do whatever you can manage. The word 'exercise' can put people off, but literally any kind of movement, whether it's slow walking through the park or gentle stretching in your living room, makes a difference.

Your mouth

Many chemotherapy drugs for breast cancer can cause everything from a painful, sensitive mouth (which I can only describe as feeling like you've just taken a big gulp of a far-too-hot coffee) to ulcers and sores inside your mouth.

My oncologist prescribed soluble co-codamol that I could use as a mouthwash to relieve them. And, on the advice of someone on Instagram, I found that keeping my mouth as clean as possible helped keep the ulcers at bay – brushing and flossing after every meal, with a soft toothbrush so as not to aggravate your gums. Spicy food was off the menu for me during chemo, as even a very moderate curry felt like fire in my mouth.

Nausea and vomiting

This is one of the most commonly reported side effects, but modern anti-sickness medication means it's nowhere near as bad as it used to be. The only time I actually vomited was after the first cycle when I didn't take the drugs that they'd given me to have at home. However, I did experience near-constant nausea.

If you've ever been pregnant, you may notice lots of parallels with cancer treatment: the fatigue, the endless blood tests and the relentless nausea that can only be eased by eating. Oh my goodness, the eating. I ate so much during chemo, not only because it helped when I felt sick but also because the steroids make you hungry. So I would advise you to fill your kitchen with healthy comfort foods. I will go into more detail about nutrition in Part III, but what I'll say for now is: if you're going to eat a lot, you might as well get the veg in. My favourites during chemo were hearty warming meals that didn't hurt my mouth: vegetable lasagne, fish pie, lentil bolognese, bean-based casseroles, Thai salmon with noodles, veggie shepherd's pie, sweet potato tray bake, and mild chickpea curry.

You might have read that fasting around chemo infusions can improve outcomes, and there is a certain amount of evidence supporting this, but don't put any pressure on yourself. I didn't know about the benefits of fasting at the time and, even if I had, I'm not sure I could have restricted my eating when I felt so queasy. If you personally feel that fasting is doable and effective on chemo days, then go for it. But please don't feel as though you have to.

One thing that I normally love but couldn't face during chemo was coffee, which exacerbated the nausea. So, instead of coffee, I got into the habit of boiling up fresh ginger in a large pan of water, then decanting it into bottles to keep in the fridge and drink throughout the week. I found this helped so much with the nausea that I was able to reduce my anti-sickness pills as the weeks went on.

Peripheral neuropathy

This common side effect is a condition affecting the peripheral nerves, which are the ones closest to the surface of the skin. These can often be damaged by certain chemo drugs, including paclitaxel, docetaxel and carboplatin. The symptoms of peripheral neuropathy can include a feeling of pins and needles or tingling, usually in the hands or feet, and, paradoxically, a sense of numbness *and* a burning or shooting pain. You may also find fiddly tasks such as tying shoelaces or doing up buttons difficult. If you experience this, tell your oncologist right away as they will want to keep a close eye on you. Sadly, there is not much you can do about it. However, in most cases, including mine, it can feel quite uncomfortable towards the end of treatment but improves quite rapidly once chemo is over. Be aware too that it can become quite serious and last for a long time, so if yours is becoming debilitating, discuss reducing the dose or frequency of treatment.

Palmar-Plantar Erythrodysesthesia

Also known by the catchier name of Hand-Foot Syndrome, this was a side effect that I experienced while taking capecitabine, a drug given as adjuvant chemotherapy. It bizarrely causes red, painful soles of your feet and palms of your hands. I found it manageable for the first few cycles, with diligent moisturising (using a simple fragrance-free product like Weleda or Aveeno), but it did become quite debilitating towards the end. I was on it for around six months and, if it had gone on for any longer, I would have had to reduce my dose as it was preventing me from walking any distance and making normal daily activities quite difficult. Wearing soft socks and slippers around the house helped – as well as having someone around to help me open jars and bottles.

Dry eyes

This also affected me while on capecitabine, but there are several chemo drugs that can cause it. I'm slightly short-sighted and have a pair of glasses that I only really use for driving. However, while on capecitabine, my eyesight deteriorated to the point that I could barely see, even with my glasses on. This confused my oncologist initially but, after a referral to an ophthalmologist, I was told this is actually pretty common. My eyesight was being affected by what he described as 'extreme dry eyes'. It was partly a side effect of the chemotherapy and partly a result of chemo having pushed my body into early menopause (which causes dryness everywhere, it seems). The experience made me feel anxious, vulnerable and utterly destabilised. I was given Hycosan Extra eye drops, which you can buy over the counter and helped me a lot. And the situation rapidly improved once I'd finished my course of capecitabine.

Your skin

I can't go into every single side effect of chemotherapy (you've seen the list they hand out when you sign the consent form). But I have to include this one as dry, painful skin is commonly reported during chemotherapy.

It didn't hit me too badly, perhaps because I'm already someone who is diligent about staying hydrated and moisturising my skin. Use a very simple, unfragranced moisturiser. Weleda worked well for me and, for more advice on what products are safe and effective, do check out The C-List, an online beauty and wellness platform for anyone going through cancer treatment. They sell everything from natural moisturisers and oils suitable for use during chemo or radiotherapy, to false eyelashes and sleep sprays. They also share videos showing how to do everything from tie a headscarf to apply false eyelashes. It's great for those little things that will help you feel a bit more 'together', if that's what you need right now.

Anything you can do to look after yourself during this time is going to help you feel better able to cope. What that looks like for you might be very different to the next person with the same diagnosis. For example, some people feel psychologically better if they wear make-up and smarter clothes, whereas others prefer to go low-maintenance in trusty old track pants. Some people feel calm when they know they're nourishing themselves with healthy food, and they enjoy buying seasonal vegetables and preparing a nutritious meal – whereas others find more joy in lying on the sofa bingeing Netflix while eating comfort food that someone else has prepared. There are people who like to use the time spent in the chemo chair productively (I once saw a man join a work meeting over Zoom during his infusion!), while others want to zone out with cosy escapism in the form of a novel or a romcom.

It will be a case of finding what works for you, depending on how your body reacts to the drugs, and how you personally feel about taking so many. Because it is a real cocktail. You might find that your system tolerates all of these medications well, and there is no need not to take everything the doctor prescribes. I didn't love the idea of having medications to counteract the side effects of other medications, and felt as though my body was a toxic waste dump at some points during chemo. If you feel the same, do talk to your oncologist about other ways to soothe side effects, because it should be a conversation and a partnership.

Hair loss

Last, but certainly not least (in my case anyway), let's talk about your hair. I could write an entire book about hair loss during chemotherapy. Despite the nausea, the fatigue, and the pain and discomfort of endless needles and tests, I still maintain that losing my hair was the worst thing about it. It's not just the hair on your head of course, but your eyelashes and eyebrows too. And it's only when they go that you realise how important they are to your face. I remember looking in the mirror and feeling a heart-crushing sadness at the doughy-faced person in a headscarf that I couldn't believe was me.

There are steps that you can take to reduce hair loss, and some people even find that, although their hair thins out during chemo, they manage to hold on to most of it. So, if your hair is important to you (and I understand this is not the case for everyone), it's worth trying everything you can.

Scalp-cooling technology

I wore the cold cap to reduce hair loss, which is essentially a helmet-like device containing liquid coolant that flows through a tube at the back of your neck from a large machine. It works by cooling your scalp to reduce blood flow to your head. I canvassed opinions on social media and some people enthusiastically recommended it after retaining most of their hair, while others said it didn't work for them, and advised me not to put myself through any additional discomfort during chemo. For me, I felt the chance of keeping at least some of my hair would be worth it.

The brand used in most British hospitals is Paxman Scalp Cooling Technology and they have produced an excellent guide for patients about how to use it in the most effective way, at coldcap.com. Although it does feel rather like wearing a hat of ice, Claire Paxman, of Paxman Scalp Cooling, assures me that it does not literally freeze your head. 'It's a common misconception, but we do not freeze your hair follicles,' she explains. 'We're taking them to the optimum temperature of 18 to 22 degrees.' The reason it feels colder than that is because the liquid coolant has to be sub-zero to achieve the temperatures rapidly. 'But we've come a hell of a long way from the old type of cold caps, which were around minus-20 degrees,' she adds.

The cap must be on for at least 30 minutes before the infusion starts, throughout the process, and some time afterwards, so it does add to the time you're in the chemo chair. It comes with a strap to go under your chin and must be fitted extremely tightly, making contact with every part of your head, in order to work effectively. It's certainly uncomfortable, but the worst bit is the first 10–20 minutes. If you can get through that, then the feeling settles down into a kind of numbness or a dull ache. I found it helpful to line up a romcom on my iPad as a distraction. Sadly, I now can't watch Drew Barrymore or Sandra Bullock prat-falling into a meet-cute without remembering the feeling of my head slowly freezing over. You can also pop a couple of paracetamol 30 minutes before the cold cap is fitted, to take the edge off.

One thing to bear in mind is that making your head cold inevitably makes you cold all over. I've seen people filling up hot water bottles on the chemo ward, but a friend gave me the brilliant tip of buying a small heated pad, which I could plug in behind the chemo chair. It was about £20 from Amazon and truly made a difference to my comfort during chemo. The only thing I would say is that I developed a rash on my legs where the heated pad had been, so I'd recommend moving it around your body during the infusion as it's probably not ideal for the heat to be concentrated in one place.

Sadly, I still did lose most of my hair, but more slowly than I would have otherwise. It wasn't obvious until around two months into chemotherapy. 'Hair retention does differ depending on the type of chemotherapy and the dose,' explains Claire. She says the treatment I had (four fortnightly cycles of AC chemo, followed by 12 weekly doses of Taxol/Carbo) is some of the most hair-loss-causing types of chemo. 'But across all the chemotherapy ranges, you've got a 50 per cent chance of retaining 50 per cent or more of your hair.'

I also invested in a Manta hairbrush, which is like a very gentle version of a Tangle Teezer, created by Tim Binnington whose wife, Dani, lost her hair during breast cancer treatment. The soft and flexible brush is anti-static, reduces breakage, and was the only thing I wanted anywhere near my head during chemotherapy.

It can be the case that there is 'tenting' at the top of the cold cap, leaving a gap between the coolant and the top of your head, resulting in a Friar Tuck-style bald patch. This happened to me and, with no headscarf, the thin wisps of hair around my bald patch actually looked worse than if I had just shaved it all off. But, with my headscarf on, I liked the fact that I still had some hair to poke out the bottom – I felt it looked less cancery than a completely bald head. It's very much a personal choice.

During this time, one of the chemo nurses recommended I stop using the cold cap. She said that the exposed scalp on the top of my head could be damaged, actually inhibiting regrowth. Luckily, I insisted on continuing, brushing over my remaining hair to protect the bald bits. 'The idea that it could damage hair follicles is a myth,' says Claire, explaining that you can protect any exposed scalp by either brushing over hair as I did, or wearing a paper theatre cap.

Daniel Field is a hairdresser who has created a range of products that work in tandem with the cold cap, called the Scalp Cooling Booster System. These include a product that looks a bit like a chicken fillet, which you place inside the cold cap to reduce that tenting effect and, hopefully, prevent the bald patch. I didn't learn about these products until too late, so can't vouch for them, but lots of people swear by them.

Even if you do experience extensive hair loss, it's worth persevering with the cold cap. 'By continuing to scalp cool, even if you feel it's not worked, you are protecting your follicles to the point that hair grows back thicker and faster within a 12-week period,' Claire explains. Indeed, by the time chemo finished, I was reassured to see that my hair was already starting to grow back on top. Two months later, I ditched the headscarf in favour of hair bands and clips. Another couple of months and the shortest bits were long enough for my hairdresser to chop into a crop.

People often ask me if it was worth it. I would say that depends on many factors. First, talk to your oncologist about how likely you are to lose all of your hair, as certain types of chemo cause 'hair thinning' rather than 'hair loss'. Then, think about how important your hair is to you versus how much you want to eliminate as many elements of discomfort as possible during chemotherapy.

Headscarves and hats

Towards the end of my neoadjuvant chemotherapy, I was in this odd middle ground where I had lost too much hair to feel comfortable leaving the house without covering the bald bits, but I still had enough hair to not get a wig. Headscarves and hats were the answer.

It will take a bit of trial and error to find out what works for you, but there are plenty of videos out there demonstrating different ways to tie a headscarf. Take a look at Headwrappers and The C-List online for inspiration.

Natural fabrics are best, particularly if you're dealing with menopausal hot flushes at the same time. I would recommend getting the nicest scarf you can afford. After all, you're going to wear it a lot. A friend gave me a silk scarf from Rixo that I actually enjoyed wearing. Having said that, towards the end, when I wanted more variety, I would pick up cheapo scarves from the high street and they were completely fine.

Tying a scarf takes a bit of getting used to, but after a few weeks you'll be able to do it with your eyes closed. I also bought a silk elasticated hair wrap from a brand called Silke London. It looked a bit like a turban but was easy to slip on and off quickly.

In colder months, you can wear a beanie hat indoors and outdoors without anyone batting an eyelid. I found that easier than the headscarf, and lived in a cashmere beanie from H&M.

Wigs and extensions

If you prefer to try a wig, you should definitely look at the NHS options before you spend a lot of money on one. Those from the NHS that I saw actually looked pretty good, although they all came with a fringe to conceal the seam at the front, which is not ideal if you don't suit a fringe (I don't).

Even if you don't wear an NHS one, you don't need to spend an arm and a leg. One of things that put me off initially was that I thought, to get a natural-looking wig, it would have to be made of real hair and cost a fortune. But I have seen wigs bought from Amazon for less than £50 that look amazing. Synthetic wigs usually cost less than £200, while wigs made from real hair can cost up to £2,000, and require more maintenance in terms of washing and styling.

As a more long-term (but also more expensive) solution, many people recommend hair-loss specialist Lucinda Ellery, who has developed the Intralace System, where a breathable mesh is woven into your remaining hair and then more hair is added, disguising hair loss while it grows back underneath. This has the benefit of being on your head all the time, so you're not constantly taking off and putting on a wig. Some people consider it life-changing during chemo, but others don't like the idea of having something on their head all the time. After all, it does mean your scalp only gets a proper wash at appointments when the mesh is changed, roughly every six to eight weeks. It's also a huge time commitment, since it involves pulling each individual hair through the mesh at each of these appointments. And the price is prohibitively expensive for many people, as it can easily spiral into thousands.

HAIR LOSS TAKEAWAYS

- Do your research on the cold cap to work out if it's right for you.
- Wash your hair less often – I only did it on chemo days – and use a very gentle, sulphate-free shampoo.
- Invest in a hair brush that won't tug on your remaining hair, such as a Tangle Teezer or Manta.
- Don't give up on headscarves too soon; it takes practice and perseverance if you've never worn one before.
- If you decide to shave it all off and get a wig, don't spend a fortune on something you're only planning to wear for a few months.
- Don't be afraid to change your mind. You can start off with the cold cap, then decide not to use it and just buy a wig.

Eyelashes and eyebrows

The cold cap sadly does little to prevent losing your lashes and brows during chemo. When I was diagnosed, a friend who had been through chemo recommended I get microblading, a tattooing technique used to apply semi-permanent make-up over your eyebrows, which can last up to two years. Sadly, because it was lockdown, I wasn't able to do that before chemo started and, once you're in the swing of it, you shouldn't have any kind of tattoo because of the risk of infection. So that's something I'd recommend, although I acknowledge that organising semi-permanent make-up might not be at the forefront of your mind when you've just been handed a cancer diagnosis.

False eyelashes can be a huge help in terms of making you feel better about how you look. And you can buy natural-looking ones, so you won't look like a *Drag Race* contestant, which was my fear. I found Lola's Lashes the easiest to apply as they have tiny magnets that clip easily on to a swipe of magnetic liner. There are also topical products that you can use to encourage regrowth as soon as chemotherapy has ended. These include UKlash and Revitalash, a serum that was actually developed for chemotherapy patients.

If you're struggling with how you look during cancer treatment, please don't think that it's silly or vain to feel that way. I often felt stupid for crying about my hair, when I knew how lucky I was to be receiving life-saving treatment on the NHS. But it's a part of your identity, and feeling uncomfortable and self-conscious every time you leave the house is another burden placed on you when you're already dealing with a lot.

It was somebody in the Maggie's centre at Barts who pointed me in the direction of the charity Look Good Feel Better. They offer skincare and make-up advice to deal with the side effects of chemo, so I signed up for one of their virtual workshops, but with low expectations. At that time, I felt so desolate about my appearance, I didn't think a few make-up tips could possibly help me. What I didn't expect was for the workshop to provide the rush of understanding and support that comes from talking to people in the same boat. After two hours of chatting about brow products and post-chemo hair growth, and applying make-up in front of my laptop along with the other women on Zoom, I learned so much. Not only about how to pencil on an eyebrow where there isn't one but also about the power of beauty to make you feel better. Their workshops are free and I can't recommend them highly enough.

Your nails

I was so caught up in the fear of losing my hair that I barely gave a thought to my nails, sadly to their detriment. Chemotherapy attacks your nails and skin, causing dehydration and sensitivity, which can be extremely uncomfortable. People can suffer symptoms ranging from their fingernails turning completely black to lifting up off the nail bed and even falling off. It might first appear as a slight bruise-like colour near your cuticle, or you might notice a blueish-black vertical line down your nail.

Prevention is better than cure, so plan ahead:

- Keep your hands and nails well moisturised, with a simple fragrance-free cream or oil.
- Some chemo wards offer gel-filled cooling gloves and slippers to protect your nails, working in the same way that the cold cap protects your hair.

- There are products designed to protect nails during chemo, such as Poly Balm, which showed impressive results during a large randomised controlled trial.
- Dark nail polish is a good idea not only to disguise the effects on your nails but also to protect them, as chemo nails are incredibly sensitive to UV light.
- If you're not a fan of dark polish, a base coat or a ridge filler will give a layer of protection and a physical barrier to reinforce the nail.
- When wearing nail polish, don't assume there is no point being as diligent with moisturiser. It absorbs in around the edges and near your cuticles, so it will still support healthy growth.
- Nail polish remover can be dehydrating and, if your nails are feeling sensitive, it can make that worse. So always look for a remover without acetone, as that will be the gentlest way to remove any polish.
- You might feel cautious about the toxic chemicals in nail polish, but there are many brands these days – such as Mavala and Nail Kind – that are made with more natural ingredients.
- Gel nails and acrylics – particularly the removal of them – can strip the natural oil out of the nail so should be avoided during chemotherapy.
- In fact, it's better to avoid nail salons during this time because of the risk of infection, so invest some time in taking care of your nails at home.

As your healthy nails grow back after chemotherapy, keep them in good condition by regularly moisturising and keeping them short and neat to prevent ingrowing nails or infections. It is partly the massaging action, as well as the actual product, that will help support strong nail regrowth.

Do remember your feet too, and avoid walking around barefoot to reduce your risk of damaging the skin and causing an infection. I suffered from discoloured fingernails during chemotherapy, although luckily I didn't lose any of them, and they seemed to grow back quite quickly after treatment. My toenails on the other hand . . . I thought they hadn't been affected by treatment at all because they seemed fine. Then, six months after my neoadjuvant chemo had finished, I stubbed my toe and my big toenail came clean off. My oncologist explained that, since toenails grow more slowly than fingernails, the effects take longer to reveal themselves. So take good care of your feet for at least six months after chemo.

Don't underestimate the confidence-boosting impact of keeping your nails in good condition. It's similar to when people talk about 'the lipstick effect' as a psychological support in tough times. Those little things are more powerful than you think.

Staying positive during chemotherapy

Yes, sorry, I'm saying the P word. One thing that I hated during active cancer treatment was people telling me to 'stay positive'. It made me feel as though I was failing because I felt anxious, frightened and utterly bereft as my hair fell away from my head in clumps. But, according to breast cancer oncologist Professor Peter Schmid, doctors and patients both spend so much time dwelling on the downsides and the negative effects of chemotherapy, that we almost lose sight of why we're doing it in the first place – which is clearly to give us the best chance of being cured.

'I'd like to bring the focus back onto why we are doing this,' he says. 'Obviously, this is not going to be an easy time for patients, but they are very much aware of the fact that there will be side effects, and we can manage them and get the patients through this together, as a team. For me, positive energy is really important.'

Professor Schmid suggests using visualisation as a powerful tool to reframe your experience. If you find that you are really suffering from the side effects of chemotherapy, take time to imagine how the cancer cells are suffering even more. Visualising your tumour actually shrinking as the chemo does its thing is an excellent way to support your emotional wellbeing. 'It's an unpleasant therapy, but cancer is not pleasant,' he continues. 'It's something we need to deal with. So chemotherapy is a fantastic opportunity. It's something positive that you're doing to help cure your body of cancer.'

I would add a caveat here, for anyone who is not going through treatment themselves but is looking for ways to support a loved one: this mindset change will not work if suggested by you. Even when framed in the best possible way, it's still a really difficult thing to go through. A person receiving chemotherapy will not be delighted to have someone with no personal experience of it telling them how great it is. If you've ever given birth, think of how it feels when a man tells you what a beautiful experience you get to have.

If you are the patient, however, then this is really worth trying. Professor Schmid believes this simple mental shift can make a huge psychological difference to people going into treatment. 'Think about when you buy a car,' he says. 'If the person selling you the car told you that, actually, driving is really bad for the environment, and there's a small risk that you might be involved in an accident and become paralysed or perhaps lose a leg. Also, you might kill a child. Would you buy that car? Probably not.'

You might be rolling your eyes at that analogy, because buying a car is clearly different to starting chemo, but your approach and attitude to something can hugely affect your experience of it. Oncologists have to make sure that you clearly understand the side effects of any new treatment, of course they do. But could they couch it in a slightly more positive way?

'We take informed consent very seriously, and rightly so,' says Professor Schmid. 'But it should be a balance of information, of the pros and cons. I'm not sure, as oncologists, we are always that balanced. We can cause a lot of fear and anxiety by focusing on the negatives. It's part of our responsibility to get positive energy in there, too. And that's where I don't think that we always do an optimal job. It's very difficult to go through chemotherapy without that feeling of hope.'

Staying active

Research has shown that being active during chemotherapy enables the optimal dosage of chemo to be better tolerated. But there can be many barriers to getting your body moving when going through chemotherapy.

You're likely to feel absolutely exhausted during treatment. Having said that, movement is one of the best ways to improve your energy levels so, if you can face it, do it.

There might be a fear of knocking your PICC line, straining on the muscles and skin around it, or getting it sweaty, which could lead to infection. The key is to go gently, and listen to your body. Now that I follow lots of cancer accounts on Instagram, I often see people running or lifting weights with a PICC line in their arm. But it's unlikely they went straight to doing that from a sedentary starting point. Find what feels comfortable for you, then slowly build it up.

There are specific yoga-for-cancer classes that you can do online or in person. Talk to local cancer groups to find one, pop into your local Maggie's centre, or call the helpful team at Breast Cancer Now, who will be happy to point you in the right direction. Yoga teacher Vicky Fox's book, *Yoga for Cancer*, shows how the practice can ease many symptoms of cancer treatment.

If you're in London, Future Dreams House in King's Cross has regular yoga, strength and even ballet classes for anyone affected by breast cancer. Look at their website to book online. Most classes cost only an optional donation.

Walking is easy, free and good when anything else feels like just too much.

I was certainly anxious about my PICC line, and it put me off any kind of exercise. I didn't know then what I know now about the statistics, showing that movement improves outcomes so much that in other countries, including Australia, it is prescribed alongside cancer treatment. At the time, I assumed rest was the most important thing. Of course, rest is important but, looking back, I wish I'd made more of an effort to move my body. Not only is it vital for keeping you strong during chemo, it can also reduce your risk of recurrence.

So make sure you're doing some form of movement, no matter how gentle. Find something that you can easily incorporate into your life. And don't think of it (or, indeed, any of the advice in this book) as something that works in a vacuum. It must be a part of wider lifestyle choices that will help support your immune system and build your neutrophils back up in between chemo sessions. All the elements work together anyway. For example, finding ways to manage stress is important for a healthy immune system, and the stress-relieving power of movement is well documented, too. Therefore, as well as helping you be in the best physical shape to cope with chemo, exercise also has enormous benefits for your mental wellbeing. Think of this as one (albeit very important) part of a much larger whole.

Radiotherapy

You'll generally find that radiotherapy is one of the last stops on the active treatment pathway for primary breast cancer, after chemotherapy and/or surgery. Although it happens before adjuvant treatments such as tamoxifen or capecitabine.

This is one area where I had no idea what to expect: Will it hurt? How long does it take? Will it make me radioactive, like the tracer that they inject during the bone scan?

To explain it, I asked Jo McNamara and Naman Julka-Anderson, both experienced therapeutic radiographers and co-hosts of the brilliantly named Rad Chat podcast. 'Radiotherapy is the use of very high ionising radiation, so it's much more powerful than your standard X-ray that you might have in A&E for a broken bone,' explains Jo. 'It's designed to target the DNA of cancer cells. Unfortunately, radiotherapy isn't sophisticated enough to differentiate between healthy cells and cancer cells, so it will destroy both. But normal cells are able to reproduce and repair themselves whereas, with cancer cells, as soon as they're damaged, that will cause cell death, known as apoptosis.'

This is one of the reasons why radiotherapy is so draining. People often dismiss it as a breeze compared to chemo, but it can be exhausting. 'When cancer cells are damaged by radiation, they break down into dead cells, but then they need to be removed and that takes quite a lot of energy,' Naman explains. 'The other mechanism is that, when healthy cells are damaged, they need to regenerate, and that also takes a lot of energy. Your body is working hardest around six hours after your radiation dose, and then there's the cumulative effect by the end of treatment and for around two to three more weeks. We say it peaks around 10 to 14 days afterwards, but tiredness and fatigue can continue for up to six weeks, because your body is recovering.'

It happens over a shorter period of time than your course of chemo, but it's quite intense. I had 15 sessions of radiotherapy, which took place every weekday for three weeks. The actual treatment is quick, less than 30 minutes, although you may be in hospital for considerably longer as, anecdotally at least, they're often not running to schedule. You may be asked to hold your breath at certain points during the treatment.

Happily, though, it's totally painless. The other good news is that the radiation goes in and out of the body, so there is no residual radioactivity hanging around afterwards.

The practicalities

It can be scary when you first arrive, because radiotherapy departments always seem to be down in a bunker, behind several big lead doors. But actually everyone that works there is lovely. They even let me film the process on my phone once, so that I could share it on Instagram. While the radiotherapy machine looks imposing, the reality of it is that it's pretty comfortable, particularly compared to other cancer treatments. I'd rather lie in a radiotherapy machine any day, than sit in a chemo chair with a cold cap on my head.

You will be naked from the waist up, under a hospital gown, which they will remove to mark up your body with pen before each session. They cover you again during the actual treatment. Make sure you don't wear any metal jewellery.

Since it was the part of cancer treatment that I knew least about, I was pretty shocked when I turned up for my pre-treatment scan and was told that they would be tattooing little permanent marks onto my body, in order to line up the radiotherapy equipment at each session. The tattoos are tiny: literally a dot on either side of my ribs and one on my chest in between my boobs. But it hurt, because they use a blob of ink and a wiggled needle. I have two actual tattoos that hurt less. And it would have been nice to know in advance that I'd leave the hospital that day with some new ink.

I asked Jo McNamara why they don't use semipermanent tattoos. After all, it seems crazy that a dot from three weeks of radiotherapy will last longer than my painstakingly applied micro-bladed eyebrows (a procedure that uses semipermanent ink). She explained that everyone has different skin, so there is a concern that semipermanent ink might not take on all skin types. 'The future is surface guided radiation therapy,' she says, describing a new technique that uses 3D technology for precision accuracy. Although you are more likely to see this in private settings than on the NHS at this stage. 'It is much more expensive,' she admits. 'But it has seen really positive results and it's what departments are shifting to.'

I wish that had happened in time for my treatment, because the tattoos look a bit like someone has jabbed me in the chest with a black ballpoint pen. The ones on either side of my ribs are less visible, so I don't really mind them, but the one on my chest is a daily reminder of what I've been through. So I was delighted when the cosmetic tattooist who I booked to do my nipple said that she could add some brown ink over it, making it look like a mole. If you're going in for an areola tattoo, ask if they can do that while you're there, as it takes a second and erases one of the marks of cancer. Alternatively, some health trusts offer removal of radiotherapy tattoos, so do ask if that could be an option for you.

Overall, you will probably find that radiotherapy is one of the easier parts of your treatment. As a cancer patient, it's almost a treat to have an appointment where no one is jabbing you with needles (other than the initial tattoos). I don't know if I'd go as far as to say it's relaxing but, depending on where your treatment takes place, you might have chilled-out music playing. I have even heard people say they use it as an opportunity to meditate. That's a sensible approach, and a far better use of your brain than fretting about your to-do list, which is what I did.

I know that lots of people – me included – are initially resistant to the idea of radiotherapy. I thought that my treatment would be over after surgery, and I'd been through so much, I really did feel as though I couldn't cope with anything else. Again, this is to do with patient information. As someone with a triple negative tumour that had spread to several lymph nodes, I was always going to need radiotherapy, but they didn't tell me about it until I was at my lowest ebb after chemo and surgery. It felt like being kicked when I was down. I actually know people who turned down radiotherapy because they just couldn't face it. I wish it had been explained to me from the beginning, and also that they had couched it in a more positive way. Obviously, they went in with their list of side effects but, actually, no one explained to me exactly why it's important.

When your breast surgeon removes the tumour, they do their very best to clear the margins, but there is always a chance there could be some cells left behind in the breast or around the scar. 'It only takes one active cell to be left behind,' says Jo. 'And radiotherapy is a great treatment to mop them up.' This is the kind of statement that clinical oncologists should lead with, rather than their list of doom.

WHAT TO ASK YOUR CLINICAL ONCOLOGIST OR CONSULTANT THERAPEUTIC RADIOGRAPHER

- What percentage benefit does radiotherapy offer in my case?
- Do I need to have the tattoos, or do you have surface guided radiation technology?
- What can I do at home to put myself in the best place to tolerate radiotherapy well, e.g. exercise, skincare?
- What creams do you recommend I use on my skin during radiotherapy treatment?

Side effects

When I tell Jo and Naman how I couldn't get my arm above my head on the radiotherapy table initially, because of cording, they both roll their eyes with frustration. While it's great that I got referred to a physiotherapist and the issue was resolved, it should never have reached that stage.

'We're passionate about the fact that patients should get prehabilitation advice before surgery, to prevent arm mobility issues,' says Jo. 'Not just for radiotherapy but for life.' This is particularly important because radiotherapy can exacerbate mobility issues in the affected area, so staying active is vital.

We should also be warned about the fact that radiotherapy can make lymphoedema worse. 'That's because of the inflammation that the radiotherapy causes,' explains Naman. 'If there is any kind of fluid build-up, it can't move as much, so then that can cause lymphoedema. Surgery is where the risk starts, but we'll make it a bit worse. Ideally, as soon as the lymph nodes are taken out, everyone should have their arm measured for fluid levels and then monitored, but they don't unfortunately.'

The other long-lasting side effect is something that can occur years, or even decades, later. 'Radiation affects every single cell in the treatment area, and so people can end up with radiation fibrosis years later,' says Jo. 'If it happens 20 years later, people don't actually realise it's a side effect of radiotherapy. They say, "I was never told about this," but the consent form does list every single side effect. It's just, who really reads all the small print when you've been told you need treatment for cancer? If patients knew what to look out for then it would save a lot of time in terms of diagnosis, and it would also save a lot of stress because people often start to worry that it's a sign of secondary breast cancer.'

All this talk of long-term health problems sounds scary initially but, actually, radiotherapy is far less likely to cause serious issues when used to treat breast cancer. Decades-later difficulties seem to occur more often with radiotherapy to the groin area, which can cause bladder control issues down the line. For those of us having radiotherapy for breast cancer, post-radiation fibrosis generally presents as tightness or pain, making movement difficult. Radiotherapy unfortunately is the gift that keeps on giving in this respect, and it's yet another reason why movement is so important.

The problem, again, is lack of information given to patents. 'Other healthcare professionals don't really know what radiotherapy is, either,' says Jo, with a wry laugh. 'Clinical nurse specialists have a better insight, but some of them have never even entered a radiotherapy department. It's crazy, because they're meant to be supporting you. If patients can be informed about what is to come later on, that could really help in terms of doing the exercises and preparing the skin. That can be preventative, which is so important because it's a lot harder to treat these things after you've had radiotherapy.'

You can also call your radiotherapy department any time post-treatment if you have any issues or questions.

As with all forms of cancer treatment, your attitude and mindset towards radiotherapy is key. It can be easy to lean into everyone's assumption that you're very ill and frail during treatment. I remember one radiotherapy nurse asking about my plans for the rest of the day and, when I replied that I was working, she looked astonished. Admittedly, my job is sitting around tapping at a laptop, so it's almost always manageable. But there often seems to be this assumption that cancer is the only thing in your life. Don't let that be the case.

Skin

The most common and immediate side effect is the impact on your skin. This can vary dramatically, so some people may have a slight change in their skin tone, while others might have painful broken skin. 'From the first dose, there will be pinkness or redness if you have lighter skin and, if you have dark skin, the area will go darker first,' says Naman. 'The skin can start to break down so it looks more like a wound. Eventually, if it's lighter skin, it will become almost like a tan. Darker skin usually goes back to normal but, if the skin has broken down, it will result in looking a bit lighter than the original skin tone.'

There is plenty that you can do to minimise skin damage and it's worth the effort because, if left unchecked, it can be permanent. Wear loose-fitting clothing made of natural fibres such as cotton during the weeks of treatment, and protect the affected area from extremes of heat or cold, so no hot baths or cold-water swimming. In fact, all swimming should be avoided as chlorine could irritate the skin, too. Gently pat your skin dry after the shower, rather than rubbing. Some people like to keep moisturiser in the fridge to instantly cool inflamed skin. However, if the skin is broken don't put any cream on it unless specifically advised by someone in your treatment team.

Keeping the skin well hydrated is key, and your radiotherapy nurse might give you a list of approved creams to use, because many body moisturisers include fragrances that can irritate the skin. I used Aveeno and Weleda, and my skin tolerated radiotherapy well. Others that come recommended by doctors include Epaderm, Aquaphor and Flamigel. And there's a brand named MooGoo (so called because it was developed from the cream applied to cows' udders, but don't let that put you off) that sells an oncology care pack including moisturiser, a gentle cleanser, lip balm and natural deodorant.

Radiotherapy makes your skin extremely sensitive, so you'll be advised to stay out of the sun as much as possible. This is not ideal if, like me, you're a sun-worshipper and your radiotherapy happens to take place in August. I assumed the guidance would be to wear sunblock every day but, surprisingly, Naman actually advises against it. 'Normally I'd agree, everyone should be wearing sunscreen all year round,' he says. 'But during radiotherapy, we advise that you just keep the area covered because lots of sun creams have metallic elements in them, which actually makes the skin rash worse.'

And it's not only SPF that you have to worry about; lots of moisturisers and other toiletries include harsh chemicals and metals. 'There are even some creams on the market that promote themselves for use during radiotherapy, but they have metals in them,' says Jo. 'And that essentially means tiny little bits that will react to the X-rays and actually produce almost secondary X-rays. It will increase the dose to your skin surface.'

'Quite a few creams use zinc as a stabiliser,' adds Naman. 'The guidelines are still being debated, and everyone's different. Even something like E45, there's been evidence that some people have allergic reactions to it,' he says. 'If you've been using the same cream on your skin for 20 years, that clearly works for you, so there is no point changing it for radiotherapy treatment. Introducing a new agent to the skin could cause a skin rash anyway. I'd suggest sticking to what you've been using and, if you experience irritated skin during radiotherapy, then you can change it.'

So if radiotherapy is part of the treatment plan for you, now you know how important it is to be diligent with moisturiser and post-surgical exercises to reduce your risk of cording and lymphoedema. With those really simple steps, you can get through radiotherapy with your skin, and sanity, intact.

RADIOTHERAPY TAKEAWAYS

- Drink lots of water to keep your body hydrated throughout treatment, as this will help with cell renewal and protect your skin.
- Use an unfragranced moisturiser regularly on the targeted area, and ensure it's one that doesn't contain metals.
- Remember no metal jewellery at all; even small things that you might not think of, such as a wedding band or ear studs.
- See if you can tie in your hospital trips with something fun. I found a brunch place near my hospital and ended up spending a fortune on eggs and avocados during those three weeks.
- Remember you'll feel very tired for up to six weeks after treatment, with fatigue peaking 10-14 days later, so go easy on yourself.

Hormone Therapy

About 80 per cent of breast cancers are oestrogen receptor positive (ER+) and/or progesterone receptor positive (PR+), meaning that the tumour is made of cells that express receptors for those hormones. So ER+ tumours rely on the presence of oestrogen in order to keep multiplying. It might help to think of oestrogen as the petrol that fuels the cancer's engine. Hormone therapies, otherwise known as endocrine treatments, are very effective, and work by lowering levels of oestrogen in the body or blocking the oestrogen receptors on the cancerous cells.

The drugs that you will hear about most often in this context include tamoxifen and raloxifene, which are from a group of drugs known as selective oestrogen receptor modulators (or SERMs). Then there is anastrozole, exemestane and letrozole, which are aromatase inhibitors. These drugs are generally given daily in pill form.

You might also be prescribed Zoladex, an implant the size of a grain of rice, which is administered by injection into your stomach every month.

All of the above is adjuvant treatment, after surgery and/or chemotherapy, with the aim of killing any remaining cancer cells that may still be floating around in the body looking for a new place to make a tumour.

As breast cancer oncologist Professor Peter Schmid explains: 'I often say to patients, your body may like oestrogen, but it doesn't need it. Your cancer cells need that oestrogen to survive. And so these treatments give us an opportunity to kill those cancer cells and increase the chance of being cured.'

But these are not drugs that you take for a few months, like my adjuvant capecitabine. Women are usually put on tamoxifen for 10 years. 'Many years ago, we used to prescribe tamoxifen for two years,' explains Professor Schmid. 'Then we did trials comparing five years with two years and we learned that we can cure more patients. And then we did trials of 10 years versus five years, and we realised that we can cure even more patients. So these treatments work over a long period of time.'

But, he goes on, they obviously do have side effects. 'And they're very different compared to chemotherapy, where the side effects are well described. There are around three or four big side effects of chemo that almost everyone has, but they're there for a limited period of time, and that makes them more tolerable to some degree. We could all grit our teeth for a short period of time to get through something. But when it comes to several years, then we need to make difficult decisions about benefits of treatment and quality of life.'

Side effects

Hormone-related symptoms are notoriously tricky to pinpoint and describe, as they can range from anxiety or insomnia to loss of concentration or brain fog. These are all things that could be attributed to the stress of a breast cancer diagnosis or other elements of cancer treatment. And then there are some very personal, intimate symptoms that can be hard to discuss with anyone, let alone a man in a white coat.

'When you think about menopause, everyone first thinks about hot flushes, because that's obviously very well established,' says Professor Schmid. 'But there are plenty of other side effects that are less well defined. Then there is the impact on how a woman may feel as a woman, and side effects that doctors and patients both often struggle to talk about, such as vaginal dryness and libido. So these endocrine side effects can be extremely wide ranging.'

Even if you are postmenopausal before your breast cancer diagnosis, you may find that you experience these symptoms all over again. Yes, a 'second menopause' is one of the unexpected joys of breast cancer treatment. 'What I often say to patients is, when you are premenopausal, your oestrogen is here,' says Professor Schmid, raising his hand high in the air. 'During menopause, it goes down to here,' he continues, moving his hand down to shoulder height. 'And what hormone therapy does is it takes your oestrogen levels down to here.' His hand drops down out of view.

Not only is it such an enormous drop, but another one of the reasons that the side effects of a drug like tamoxifen can be so severe compared with a naturally occurring menopause is because it happens so suddenly. It's a huge shock to your system, which doesn't have time to adjust.

'And that's a really important point,' says Professor Schmid, 'because natural menopause, in many women, is a process of months and years as the endocrine function of the ovaries gradually decreases. It's not a switch-on-and-off thing.

Whereas, with our treatments, it is a pretty abrupt situation and the speed of that change certainly has an impact on how these symptoms are experienced.'

He compares it to walking into a hot room, out of the cold. You'll notice that temperature difference much more than if you were in a room that was being gradually heated, giving your body time to adjust to the new temperature. It's little wonder that many breast cancer patients want as much information as possible so that they can weigh up the benefits of the treatment versus the risk of not taking it. Professor Schmid tells me that 'life is about taking risks' and that's true, but arguably deciding whether a treatment might save your life or destroy the quality of it is the kind of risk most of us don't have to face very often. How does he advise people in that situation?

'What I've learned over the years is to try and avoid describing anything as high risk or low risk, or large benefit or small benefit because, actually, it's very individual,' he says. 'I've had patients where chemotherapy for them would mean an increased survival benefit of 1 per cent, and they are keen to do it. But I've seen other patients where a certain treatment will give them a 10–20 per cent survival benefit, and they don't feel that's worth it. The benefit comes down to the individual's perspective and where they are in life. The risk they are therefore prepared to take is linked with their personal perception of the benefit.'

After having been through cancer treatment, many of us feel as though we would do absolutely anything to avoid being in that position again. But, depending on how severely the side effects are impacting your life, you may be more inclined to weigh up the risk. If you are risk-averse in general, or particularly worried about recurrence, then you're probably prepared to accept more side effects of endocrine therapy. But it's difficult to know exactly how you personally will cope with the persistence and duration of these side effects until you're actually doing it.

'Oncologists like myself will say, "Oh, this treatment is really well tolerated compared to chemotherapy", and that's probably right in terms of the big, acute side effects,' admits Professor Schmid. 'But actually the impact on quality of life can be substantial, and that's often a difficult discussion. I spend probably more time discussing these things than any other aspect of care and, in this context, we often talk about percentages as well. Because, again, something I had to learn over the years is that a not insignificant number of women will not take endocrine therapy because of the impact on quality of life. Everyone is different, but what I can do is share my experience from listening to other patients in a comparable situation. But then they still have to work out how they feel.'

Explore all options with your oncologist, because you can always switch brand, or try another type of drug. This will be a case of trial and error, as everyone reacts differently.

As with menopausal symptoms in general, there are lifestyle steps that you can take to ease the side effects, to an extent. Exercising, managing stress, eating well and getting good quality sleep can help with some of the symptoms (see Part IV for more on this). For others, you may need further support. Comedian Jennifer Saunders revealed in 2022 that she took an antidepressant to cope with feelings of anger while on tamoxifen. And many women describe emotional symptoms including rage, as well as fear, anxiety, low mood and a debilitating brain fog that hugely affects your memory and concentration. I go into all of these symptoms more fully in Part III.

Helen's story

Helen Addis was 39 when she was diagnosed with ER+ breast cancer in 2018. She had a mastectomy first, followed by chemo and radiotherapy, and targeted treatments because her tumour was also HER2+ (more on this in the next chapter). Then she was prescribed tamoxifen, which thrust her into menopause and caused many symptoms you might associate with that, such as hot flushes. However, she struggled most with fatigue and the cognitive side effects of the drug.

'Sometimes I couldn't even string sentences together, I just couldn't find the words,' she says. As a TV producer, she manages a team, and it wasn't long before the side effects started impacting her work. 'It was so apparent to me because I was so used to having to remember a lot of stuff,' she continues. 'I really had to be across everything and I would just forget the most basic things. It did really get me down and it definitely affected my confidence. I felt everybody was looking at me like I was a complete nutter. I feel like they probably still do. And it's a vicious circle because then you feel crap about yourself, which makes it worse.'

Like many women in her situation, Helen is torn between being grateful for the treatment that made her cancer-free, and struggling with the side effects of that treatment. 'Tamoxifen is pretty much a wonder drug,' she says now. 'I am super grateful that it exists, and maybe I just have to suck it up. But also you've got to think about quality of life. So I asked if I could have a break from it and my oncologist said, "You can have a break, but do you want to risk it?" Because my cancer was very hormone sensitive. So I did have a break from tamoxifen for four weeks, and I have to say that I didn't notice much of a difference. I'm told that, had I had a longer break, I would have seen more of a difference, but I don't know that I could take that risk, so I went back on it.'

Since her diagnosis and treatment, Helen has thrown herself into campaigning work, notably with the hugely successful Change & Check campaign, which has seen stickers put on mirrors in high street changing rooms all around the UK, reminding women to check their breasts. And she's co-founder of The C-List, the beauty and wellness platform for anyone going through cancer treatment. She also shares information on her Instagram @TheTittyGritty. To an outsider, it looks as though she's always positive, and a worthwhile purpose has emerged out of her experience. But the reality is that she has found it as hard as any of us.

'The hardest part comes at the end of it all,' she says, 'because you're like, "Oh, did that just happen? That bus actually nearly hit me." It was the mental side of it, as well as everything that's going on with you physically.' She tried having counselling, through the NHS, but didn't click with the counsellor so found it hard to open up. She also makes an effort to follow all the lifestyle advice that has been shown to make a difference, such as exercising and eating well. But she has found the thing that works best for her is reiki. 'I found it really enlightening and very powerful actually,' she says. 'If you can get a good reiki master, I'd recommend that in a heartbeat.'

Her biggest piece of advice, though, is to accept all offers of help. 'People around you love you and they want to help you, so when they're offering to pick up your kids or come and put the vacuum cleaner around your house, they genuinely mean it. If the shoe was on the other foot, you'd probably be the sort of person that would want to go and do the same for them,' she says. 'You don't have to do it on your own.'

Physical effects

While the emotional impact of tamoxifen is clearly difficult, the physical side of it should also not be underestimated. Kat Tunnicliffe, oncological physiotherapist at Perci Health, tells me that SERMs and aromatase inhibitors can cause or exacerbate everything from weak bones and weight gain, to aches and pains and pelvic floor dysfunction. 'The list is endless,' she says, 'which is why it is so important that people are properly informed of the side effects, and what their recurrence chance is if they decline, before embarking on treatment. And, if someone does decline or wants alternative opinions, they have the absolute right to do this with no judgement.'

She hears time and time again about patients who just do what they're told and regret it later. 'They learn that their chances of recurrence would have been minimal, compared to no drugs, but with maintaining a healthy weight, reducing alcohol and exercising,' she continues. 'Instead they're stuck on tamoxifen with a poor quality of life. So I definitely advocate being fully informed before consenting. Take the time to really identify how you as an individual may be affected by it.'

And this advice is not only for those whose cancer is hormone receptor positive. Everyone going through treatment for breast cancer needs to consider the effect on their hormones. Many of us are thrust into early menopause, either by chemotherapy or by surgery. Turn to the menopause chapter (*page 169*) for detailed advice on specific symptoms.

HORMONE THERAPY TAKEAWAYS

- Don't suffer in silence. Try other drugs or switching brands to see it if feels better.
- Consider counselling, or an antidepressant, if endocrine therapy is making you feel really down.
- Ask your oncologist for specifics on the percentage benefit of each treatment, so you can make an informed decision.
- Lifestyle choices can have a huge impact on hormonal symptoms, so eat well, sleep well and move your body. I'll go into more detail on this in Part III.

Targeted Therapies

There are many different targeted therapies, all of which work in different ways, with different types of breast cancer. They are called 'targeted' because, unlike chemo or radiotherapy, they attack the cancer cells directly. These therapies might do this by blocking blood supply to the cancer, or blocking the signals that encourage the cells to multiply and divide. Some targeted treatments deliver toxic substances directly to the cells to destroy them or, as with immunotherapy, they stimulate the immune system to attack the cancer.

These drugs may be administered by infusion on the chemo ward, given by injection or taken as tablets. The Macmillan Cancer Support website has a brilliant list of targeted therapies and immunotherapy drugs, so, once you know what drug you're having, they will be able to provide exhaustive information about how each treatment works and any possible side effects. The information can be overwhelming and confusing, so don't forget you can always call their helpline, where they'll be more than happy to talk through any concerns with you.

As you know by now, the majority of breast cancers are hormone receptor positive, so should respond well to chemo and endocrine therapies. Targeted treatments tend to be most relevant for those whose breast cancer is HER2+ or triple negative. Although HER2 cancers can be (and often are) also hormone driven so, in those cases, you might have endocrine therapies as well as targeted treatments.

As I mentioned earlier, an immunotherapy drug called pembrolizumab is an example of a new targeted therapy that will revolutionise outcomes for patients with primary TNBC, reducing the risk of recurrence by 40 per cent. It wasn't available on the NHS when I was treated in 2021, but it is now.

Another of the big breakthroughs in targeted therapies, this time for HER2 breast cancers, came in the 1990s with the invention of Herceptin, a drug that is now widely used.

Leah's story

Like many people, journalist Leah Hardy had never heard of HER2 when she was diagnosed in September 2021, aged 58. She says the hardest point was after her diagnosis but before the scans to check that the cancer hadn't spread elsewhere in her body.

'I was convinced it had already spread and that I was going to die,' she says. 'I was absolutely terrified. I didn't tell my children right away because I wanted to give them as much time without being worried as possible. I knew that I'd have to be resilient to get through this – whatever happened. That doesn't mean I didn't have terrible thoughts and panic attacks. I got sleeping tablets from my doctor, which really helped. The thought that I'd have eight hours of stress-free oblivion at the end of the day was a lifesaver.'

Happily, the cancer hadn't spread beyond her lymph nodes, so she started chemotherapy ahead of surgery. Struggling to get her head around it all, she ended up watching a movie called *Living Proof*, starring Harry Connick Jr as Dr Dennis Slamon, the key scientist behind the targeted treatment Herceptin. It made her realise just what an incredible drug Herceptin is. It was only approved on the NHS for primary HER2 breast cancer in 2006. Just 20 years ago, Leah's story could have been very different.

Her tumour was grade three, so very aggressive, but her doctor explained that isn't always a bad thing when it comes to targeted therapies. 'The fact that the cells are so active means they are more easily identified,' she says. 'Think of the drug as a sniper who knows there's a terrorist in a crowd who's about to explode a bomb. If the terrorist is drably dressed, and acting unobtrusively, he's going to be hard to spot. But if he's dressed in carnival gear, singing and dancing and yelling, "I've got a bomb!" he's a lot easier to identify and pick off.'

Alongside her chemotherapy, Leah had Herceptin, plus another targeted treatment called Perjeta (which wasn't available on the NHS until 2016). And, brilliantly, had a complete response which meant her tumour had disappeared by the time she had her mastectomy, followed by radiotherapy. Then she continued to have Herceptin and Perjeta as a combined injection called Phesgo, every three weeks, for a further year. She is now cancer-free and feels healthier than ever.

Leah has also been having regular infusions of Zometa, a bisphosphonate that strengthens the bones. You may be offered this if you were post menopausal before your cancer diagnosis, or if treatment has pushed you into early menopause. Not only does it help strengthen your bones (important after menopause), it also makes them less hospitable to cancer cells, reducing your risk of recurrence. People with secondary breast cancer may also have it to treat symptoms such as bone pain. The side effects can include nausea and flu-like symptoms but, unlike chemotherapy where the side effects are cumulative so get worse over time, the body tends to adjust to Zometa and you'll feel better over the course of the treatment.

There are also more targeted treatments available for patients whose cancer has spread elsewhere in their body. A class of drugs called antibody-drug conjugates (ADCs) have been getting a lot of attention in breast cancer circles in recent years. Trodelvy is an ADC immune targeted therapy which is highly effective in buying more time for those with secondary triple negative breast cancer. Compared with chemotherapy, it's much easier to tolerate, and the drug directly attacks the tumour rather than every cell in the body. Enhertu is another ADC that works in a similar way, this time for those with HER2-low cancers.

Leah's story shows just how far we've come in less than 20 years. These targeted treatments are so effective, there is even talk that HER2+ cancers may become the first curable type of secondary breast cancer. 'Don't panic,' is Leah's advice to anyone with a new diagnosis. 'New treatments have absolutely transformed outcomes for patients, and there are new and better drugs in trials all the time.'

TARGETED THERAPIES TAKEAWAYS

- Ask your doctor about bisphosphonates, like the Zometa infusion. My oncologist didn't mention it to me until I brought it up. It's only for menopausal women, so if cancer treatment has stopped your periods, they will want to be certain that you are fully menopausal.
- If you are unsure that you're being offered the very latest targeted therapies, you can always ask for a second opinion.
- But don't be overwhelmed by talk of new drugs, and don't let it make you panic that you're not receiving the best treatment. Your oncologist will be straightforward if you ask them directly.

PART III:

THE END OF TREATMENT AND THE MYTH OF THE ALL-CLEAR

Towards the end of my treatment, after I had been through chemotherapy and surgery, I asked my oncologist when I would get the 'all-clear'? She actually laughed. Apparently, the 'all-clear' is something they only say in films. In real life it's not a thing. The best you can hope for is 'no evidence of disease' (or NED), which is infuriatingly vague, and applies to that moment in time only, so merely buys you a few weeks of non-anxiety.

This is one of the most difficult points of the journey for many people. When treatment finishes, there can be a sense of being set adrift or abandoned. People often underestimate how hard it can be to cope psychologically with the open-ended way in which cancer treatment wraps up. I certainly underestimated it.

My surgeon did actually mention, just as I was finishing chemo and heading into surgery, that lots of people find it difficult when they reach the end of treatment. I remember thinking, *Why?* Why would you not just be delighted that the pain and trauma of cancer treatment is over? I was looking forward to it finishing so I could get on with my life, and didn't even consider that I would struggle emotionally. I was wrong.

Post-traumatic Stress

Everybody around you thinks, "Oh how marvellous, you've finished your treatment. Aren't you lucky? You're cured! You can go back to work as normal. You should be doing a song and dance number because it's all over,"' says Karen Verrill, centre head at Maggie's Newcastle. She has 40 years' experience as a clinician specialising in breast cancer, including 10 at Maggie's, and she runs groups with large numbers of patients with primary or secondary diagnoses, so she knows her stuff. 'It's really not over, at all,' she says. 'The impact of that diagnosis and the psychological trauma of cancer treatment can come crashing down on people.'

These feelings can come as a shock, not only to those around you, but to you yourself. And it's important to address them as soon as you can, because they can easily escalate. Nobody wants to pile more bad news on you when you've had a cancer diagnosis, so I can understand why oncologists and surgeons might feel disinclined to explain that, once treatment is over, the cognitive shock can really kick in. Symptoms can range from low mood and anxiety to full-blown depression. The feeling of separating from the healthcare system that has been keeping you alive is understandably terrifying, and psychological support services see a big increase in referrals at this time, because people are finally processing the shock and overwhelm of cancer treatment. That is why cancer care in Germany puts so much effort into what happens next. As I wept in my oncologist's office, she explained that this point, at the end of treatment, is when she most often refers people for counselling.

I once heard this post-treatment moment being compared to narrowly avoiding being hit by a bus. You jump out of the way, shaken and panicky. You don't have a little celebration at the side of the road because you're still alive. Your adrenaline and cortisol are surging, and your brain needs time to adjust from the shock. It's that feeling, on steroids. Not least because you've probably literally been on steroids.

More brutally, Karen compares finishing cancer treatment to the experience of a soldier returning from war. 'When they're in the thick of it, being bombed and shelled and shot at, they cope with it because they have to,' she explains. 'If they're going to fall apart, it's when they get home. And it's the same for women going through breast cancer. They are bombed and shelled and shot at by cancer treatment and then, when it's all over, it hits them more because they keep themselves together when it's happening. It's only when it stops that they've got time to understand what they've been through.'

Dr Nina Fuller-Shavel goes further when talking about cancer treatment and trauma. 'I'm really passionate about getting healthcare professionals to screen for trauma because actually we have a bigger prevalence of post-traumatic stress disorder among cancer survivors in the UK than we do in veterans who've seen armed conflict,' she says. Let that sink in. 'A higher percentage of cancer survivors have trauma, and it's persistent trauma because it doesn't get recognised, and it doesn't get treated properly. We do nothing about it.'

Dr Fuller-Shavel says this systemic neglect of cancer patients' trauma is particularly acute when it comes to younger people. When people are diagnosed in their 70s, by then they generally have a peer group who might have gone through cancer treatment. When you get diagnosed under 50, many people haven't known anyone diagnosed with breast cancer at their age. So, on top of the trauma of diagnosis and treatment, it's an incredibly lonely place.

'It's inertia to assume that people with cancer are going to have a really awful time and that's just the way it is,' she continues. 'Given enough support, it can be a very different experience for people.'

If you're struggling with traumatic symptoms, then don't suffer in silence. Symptoms of post-traumatic stress disorder (PTSD) include distressing recurrent flashbacks or nightmares in response to reminders of the trauma, and avoidance of distressing memories, feelings and associated triggers. You might experience hyper-vigilance, problems with sleep and concentration, as well as mood swings and detachment, emotional numbness or persistent negative beliefs. If this all feels horribly familiar, make an appointment with your GP and talk to them about a treatment specific for PTSD, such as EMDR (Eye Movement Desensitisation and Reprocessing), which is recommended by the NICE (National Institute for Health and Care Excellence) guidelines and can be made available on the NHS.

'You just need to be quite specific about what kind of therapy you need,' says Dr Fuller-Shavel, 'because often they might say, "Oh you're anxious and depressed," and they'll just send you straight into the normal stream for CBT, but that's a sticking plaster. Actual proper trauma therapy really does transform people's lives. I've seen it do that.'

If you can't face going through those channels but want to give it a go, there are videos on YouTube that explain how EMDR works, and give you a taste of it. There are also people who swear by Emotional Freedom Techniques (EFT), also known as tapping, for managing emotions. Techniques can vary, but it generally involves literally tapping parts of your face and body (on energy points, similar to acupuncture, but without the needles), while repeating certain statements to change your thinking. Again, you can find guides on YouTube, or take part in online sessions through charities like Future Dreams and Penny Brohn UK.

For some people, however, traditional therapy and CBT can be extremely helpful.

Deirdre's story

Deirdre Cooper was 39 when she was diagnosed with triple negative breast cancer. She had chemotherapy, a mastectomy and radiotherapy, finishing treatment a year after her diagnosis, after which she expected to go back to normal. But anxious thoughts that stemmed from an off-the-cuff comment by her oncologist would soon grow to be overwhelming. 'I was concerned that even after five months of chemo, there was a seven-millimetre tumour left in the breast tissue,' she says. 'My oncologist confirmed that this was not ideal and said that "only time will tell." Those words still haunt me to this day.'

How did she cope after that? 'I tried to go back to being the over-efficient, competent, conscientious people-pleaser that I was, and still am. I tried to go back to normal.' Deirdre went back to her job as a solicitor on a part-time basis but, in reality, was always available on her phone. At the same time, fear of recurrence meant that she was terrified to miss a second of her three children's lives, racing from the school gate to the office and back again. 'I was trying to be normal,' she says now. 'I was trying to prove at work that I could be like I was before. I never mentioned the C-word because I didn't want pity. I thought that I didn't need counselling, because what was it going to change? The facts were the facts, that was that.'

It wasn't until two years later, when the Covid pandemic hit, that Deirdre was forced to acknowledge that she wasn't coping. The brutal combination of home-schooling and the lack of boundaries on working hours was a challenge for many of us, but it coincided with Deirdre having an expired coil removed, resulting in an acceleration of early menopausal symptoms. Feelings of overwhelm and anxiety became relentless and, hating the thought that she wasn't coping, she tried harder. It was a vicious circle that eventually led to a breakdown.

'I couldn't sleep, was riddled with anxiety and then felt low, a type of low I had never experienced before,' she explains. 'I had to give up work, go on medication and start to try and unravel everything that had happened. I don't entirely blame early menopause. It was merely the thing that gave me that extra push, along with Covid, to break down and come to terms with everything that had happened to me. I went to counselling with a specialised former breast care nurse and that was brilliant; I finally grieved for the loss of my old life. Then I did a lot of CBT, which was helpful for giving me coping mechanisms, deep breathing being the most effective one. I finally accepted that my old normality was never going to return. I was a totally different me.'

A breast cancer diagnosis at any age is hard, but for younger patients it's often the first time they've been face-to-face with their own mortality. This can feel terrifyingly overwhelming, and many young mothers torture themselves with imagined scenarios of their children's grief if their mother died. If this is the case for you, and you thought you didn't need counselling, it might be worth looking into. There is no right or wrong way to deal with what you've been through, but some kind of therapy can help with acceptance and emotional healing. Don't expect overnight results though; this tends to be the beginning of a longer process, with many ups and downs.

Deirdre says she's now in a much better place, and able to talk about her diagnosis and treatment without feeling judged or pitied. She has a new job and is strict with her boundaries: when the laptop is closed, she's off duty. 'I am now very aware of when I need to pull back and focus on myself,' she says. 'I no longer compare myself to others, especially when it comes to the ability to cope. Just because they look like they're coping doesn't mean I have to compete. I have become less tolerant of people who don't make me feel good, and I did exit certain people from my life. Of course, I wouldn't have chosen my path at all. But now that I have travelled it, I feel so much wiser for it. I look at what people around me get fixated on and I simply laugh.'

Get support

Deirdre's story could have been much easier and simpler had she had the right support from the beginning. Once you've been through cancer treatment, you should be warned about what to expect, and be able to have a conversation with a medical professional about the warning signs, in the same way that they do with post-natal depression. I'm sure some doctors are more attuned to this than others, so you might be lucky in terms of emotional support, but you might not.

So thank goodness for organisations like Maggie's, who run a six-week course called Where Now? for people coming out the other side of cancer treatment. There are breast cancer-specific ones, so you'll be in a group with others who have finished their main treatment for breast cancer, although they may still be on an adjuvant treatment like tamoxifen, Herceptin or capecitabine.

'At the beginning of the course, they're all feeling very fragile and emotional,' says Karen, who runs the course at Maggie's Newcastle. 'They have often lost confidence in themselves, and they usually have some body image issues, as well as all the anxiety that goes with finishing cancer treatment.'

The course is run with the help of a psychologist who specialises in cancer patients and can pick up on any serious issues early on. And a personal trainer is there for every session, to make sure the participants on the course are moving their bodies every day. They will go on to talk about the benefits of movement, nutrition and emotional wellbeing, as well as post-treatment challenges and what to look out for in terms of recurrence. Then they cover ways to deal with anxiety and fear around that. But one of the most important aspects of the course is the chance to talk to other people dealing with exactly the same issues as you, and the sense of camaraderie that comes with that. 'By the end of the course it's like a hen party in there,' laughs Karen. 'Sometimes it's a hen party by week two, that's how much better they feel.'

Breast Cancer Now run a similar course called Moving Forward, which is online and so accessible to everyone, no matter where you are in the country. And Life After Cancer is an excellent organisation, running a mix of online and in-person support groups and courses.

As well as confronting your own emotional issues after treatment, it's also important to talk to those around you about how you feel – even if they don't necessarily want to hear it. 'Your relatives want you to feel well so that they can stop worrying, because watching someone you love go through cancer treatment is awful,' says Karen. 'They're desperate for you to feel better so that they can feel better. Their discomfort subsides if you're fine and happy but when that doesn't happen, they struggle to understand. You might hear them say things like, "What's wrong with you? You should be happy now. You've been so brave during the treatment, why are you like this now?" When, actually, it's more common to struggle afterwards than it is during treatment.'

You probably didn't expect to still be struggling, at this point in the process, with the most deceptively simple of questions: 'How are you?' When there are so many huge emotions flying around inside your body, it's tempting to fall back on 'fine' as a response. But I'd strongly advise you not to pretend that everything's fine when it's definitely not. That will only make you feel more pressure to put on a brave face, and right now you need to be reducing the pressure wherever you can.

Remember, you can always say, 'There are good days and bad days.' If you want to be positive, you could say something like, 'I'm very happy that chemo is over,' which swerves those post-treatment feelings without quashing them. A line that worked for me was: 'Well, my hair's growing back.' A casual acquaintance would read this as: 'My hair's growing back, so things are great.' Whereas a friend who knew me better would read it as: 'My hair's growing back, but. . .'

Fear of recurrence

This is a huge cause of anxiety for people after breast cancer treatment. If the cancer comes back, it's less likely to be in the other breast and more likely to reappear somewhere else in the body. This is known as metastasis, or secondary breast cancer, and, once this happens, the cancer is no longer curable and can only be managed. We will look at secondary breast cancer more fully in the following chapters, but it's important to say that for those of us with a primary diagnosis the fear of this happening can be overwhelming at times.

Shortly after my treatment, I had a follow-up appointment with a surgical registrar (rather than my usual surgeon) who had clearly missed the 'no scaremongering' lecture at medical school. She explained that since my cancer was triple negative, multifocal, grade three and, as I did not have a complete response to chemo, I was at high risk of recurrence. She advised me to be 'extremely vigilant', as there is every possibility that there are rogue cancer cells rooting around in my body, looking for a new place to make a tumour. Later, at a routine appointment, my oncologist said I should never have been told that.

'So it isn't true?' I asked, hopefully.

'Well, it's factually correct,' said my oncologist, 'but it doesn't help to hear it.'

After all, 'high risk' is relative, and there is still a good chance that the cancer will not come back and I'll live a long, healthy cancer-free life. Is there a way to make your brain focus on that positive outcome, while also being vigilant for signs of recurrence? Possibly, but it's certainly not easy.

People who have been through successful treatment for

primary breast cancer are not routinely offered scans, other than mammograms, on the NHS at least. This initially seems bizarre, since recurrence is more likely to occur elsewhere in your body, such as in the bones, brain, lungs or liver. A mammogram would only detect a completely new cancer in the other breast, which is statistically less likely. However, mammograms are routine on the NHS for anyone at a higher risk of breast cancer (which you are, once you've had a previous breast cancer diagnosis), so that's why they do them. And diagnostic scans such as MRI, CT or PET scans are only carried out if you are showing symptoms of recurrence. For more on those, see the chapter on secondary breast cancer (*page 214*).

The stats on survival versus mortality show that the outlook is good: 76 per cent of people diagnosed with breast cancer will live for 10 years or more and, of the quarter of patients that don't survive, it's unclear how many were diagnosed with secondary cancer initially, rather than having had recurrence after treatment for a primary diagnosis. And treatments are improving all the time. I was prescribed capecitabine as adjuvant chemotherapy, which has been shown to reduce the risk of recurrence in patients with TNBC, and is a comparatively new treatment.

Anyway, it's easy to become obsessed with stats, frantically worrying about every headache or back pain, and work yourself into such a frenzy that you wake at 4 a.m. with your brain conjuring up dark scenarios of how your kids will cope without you. Believe me, I understand exactly how debilitating that kind of anxiety can be. It happens because the human brain hates uncertainty, to the extent that research has shown it actually prefers a predictable negative outcome to an unknown one. If you feel like this, you need to find ways to manage it.

The first thing is to understand why it is happening. The

brain is not designed to make you happy; it's designed to keep you safe. That's why it automatically searches for the worst-case scenario, spiralling into thoughts that your headache could be cancer recurrence, because it's trying to protect you. I had a relentless headache when my treatment finally came to an end, but it wasn't recurrence – it was fear and anxiety leading to a tension headache. Uncertainty around recurrence inevitably increases anxiety levels and stress hormones and leads to hyper-vigilance towards sensations in the body, which can become a vicious circle.

Managing stress and anxiety is important because our emotional health clearly impacts on our physical health. Anyone who doesn't believe the mind influences our physiology should think about how they feel when they're stressed or anxious: queasy and sweaty, with a racing heart rate and maybe even chest pains or stomach cramps. You have to find ways to manually override your brain's natural, and understandable, fear. And not by trying to ignore it, which will only make it burst back out when you least expect it. Remember fear is something that not only hasn't happened yet, but might not happen at all. So, while you must acknowledge it, it doesn't help to dwell on it. Different strategies work for different people, but here's what has helped me and others too.

Practical ways to manage fear of recurrence

Worrying about every twinge? If you feel a pain that you fear could be a sign of recurrence, set a reminder for two weeks to check if it still hurts. It's only worth worrying about new pains if they are persistent, and dwelling on something like a headache or chest pain can actually make it persist.

The act of writing it down gives your brain permission to forget about it for now, and often you'll find that it then gets better. By the time the reminder pings to ask if it's still hurting, you might have totally forgotten about it. If it's still there, get it checked out. The chances are it's still nothing, but now you can tell the doctor with certainty that you've been having those symptoms for two weeks. Most breast care nurses will ask you to wait until you've been experiencing a symptom for two weeks anyway before seeing a doctor about it.

Movement has been shown to dissipate the stress hormones adrenaline and cortisol, while stimulating the production of endorphins, which can improve your mood. It also reduces your risk of recurrence, so has the added benefit of helping you feel like you're doing something positive to protect yourself in the future. Not a natural exerciser, I have experimented with personal trainers and classes to try and make it a regular habit. But what has worked best is keeping it simple. I now have a small dumbbell and a mat in the living room and, every time I have a spare 10 minutes, I do a plank, or some squats or bicep curls.

Going to an exercise class, when you have more time, means not only are you moving your body, but also you have to focus on what you're doing, which gives your brain a break from spiralling thoughts. I love Pilates, but anything from spinning to CrossFit to Zumba to bootcamp is great.

Invest in a treatment that will soothe your mind and make your body feel cared for. Some people love acupuncture, reiki or having a massage. And you don't need to spend a fortune: the teaching clinic at London's College of Chinese Medicine offers discounted appointments with students and graduates, and I found a brilliant local reflexologist who practises in the shed at the bottom of her garden.

Mindfulness and meditation can help, but should be used with caution, as those with depressive thoughts may find that it makes them worse. The way in which it helped me is by bringing my awareness to the present moment, calming my thoughts and allowing me to focus on right now. None of us knows what the future holds – we could spend all our time worrying about cancer and then be hit by a bus. One of the simplest things you can do right now to feel better is close your eyes, take a few deep breaths, and then ask yourself: 'Aside from my thoughts, am I okay?'

Journaling can be of huge benefit to some people. And there is research to show that it's helpful to commit our thoughts to paper, rather than letting anxieties rattle around chaotically in our heads. The mere act of writing down our problems can allow us to organise them more clearly. Telling the 'story' of what we're going through makes it easier for us to process. Personally, I have tried journaling and it felt like I was wallowing in my fears. Again, it's about finding what works for you.

Speak to a professional if you're really struggling with anxious thoughts. Your medical team may be able to refer you to a psychologist, and there are private practitioners that offer everything from neuro-linguistic programming (NLP) to hypnotherapy. Many people might roll their eyes at the latter option, but a friend recommended hypnosis after it helped her relax so much that it stopped the neck pain she had become convinced was cancer.

One thing that I have found useful is to think of my emotions as characters, as in the Pixar movie *Inside Out*. If you're not familiar, it's set inside the head of an 11-year-old girl called Riley, where the emotions of joy, sadness, disgust, fear and anger are all individual characters. In showing the characters working together to help Riley, you realise the importance of less pleasant emotions. Fear, after all, is only trying to keep her safe. Thinking of your feelings in this way helps you separate yourself from them and consider them rationally. Your fear is not the bad guy. It knows that recurrence is a possibility, so it seizes on every headache or back pain as something to worry about. If you take a step back, you can say: 'Hey Fear, thanks for looking out for me but, actually, that headache is probably partly dehydration, partly tiredness, partly the menopause and partly due to you getting yourself worked up. . .'

This might not work for you. The experience of moving on from cancer treatment is different for everyone. But there is one thing that's true of everybody: the process is not smooth or linear. You will have good days and bad days. Days where you can't stop crying, or are paralysed with anxiety about recurrence, and days you barely even think about it. It's about finding a balance between being vigilant about the risk of recurrence and forgetting about it enough to relax and enjoy life.

As one friend with breast cancer said to me: 'The only way you really know that your cancer hasn't returned or spread is when you die of something else.' That might sound bleak, but I actually found it freeing. Your cancer very likely will not come back and, even if it does, do you want to have spent your cancer-free time worrying about it?

'Women, in my opinion, are wonderful creatures,' says Karen. 'They are all things to all people, and they're often juggling everything. So when they're compromised by cancer treatment and they feel fatigued and low, the thing they struggle to cope with most is not keeping it together for other people. When women come into Maggie's and they're tearful, they say things like, "I need to be back to normal for everybody else." And, with the right help, we can get them back in the driving seat and off they go.'

Another thing that people often experience when coming out the other side of treatment for primary breast cancer is almost a sense of guilt about still being scared of recurrence. We're the lucky ones, after all, and I'm sure anyone with secondary breast cancer would happily take fear of recurrence over their own situation any day. But all feelings are valid and just because you have lived to tell the tale, doesn't mean that everything in your life is perfect.

The end of cancer treatment is almost always the beginning of something else. What that 'something else' is is up to you. You have to take control of the rebuilding process, otherwise you can easily drift into fear or anxiety. Once you've had cancer, it will always be a part of your identity, but it need not define you. Importantly, we have to let go of the idea of getting back to normal, as much as that's what we'd love to do. 'Normal' is no longer a thing for us. But you can rebuild yourself post-cancer, and you might even find that normal is overrated anyway.

Menopause-related Symptoms

The word 'menopausal' is thrown around a lot, so you might be surprised to learn that 'the menopause' is actually one day. It's the day on which you haven't had periods for one year. After that, you are post-menopausal. Before that day, even when struggling with symptoms associated with the menopause, you are premenopausal or perimenopausal.

If you are already postmenopausal at the time of diagnosis, you may even find that you experience menopause-related symptoms all over again – and maybe even some new ones that you didn't have when you went through it the first time.

If you are premenopausal at diagnosis, then cancer treatment may thrust you pretty abruptly into menopause. This can happen either as a result of medical menopause, for example, chemotherapy damaging your ovaries, or with adjuvant endocrine therapies such as tamoxifen. Or it could be surgical menopause, if you have been found to have one of the breast and ovarian cancer gene mutations, so have chosen to have your ovaries removed.

The symptoms of menopause can be quite brutal, and they are incredibly wide-ranging, so you might not realise, for instance, that your insomnia or irritability are caused by your body being forced abruptly into menopause.

The difficulty in getting the right support for these issues is that so many menopause-related symptoms can be partly attributed to other things. For example, weight gain could be due to the menopause, or it could be because of the steroids you took during chemo, or the stress that you're under, or the impact that cancer treatment has had on your gut microbiome. Depression and anxiety are such common symptoms of the menopause that one in four women are prescribed antidepressants by their doctor when they should be prescribed HRT. But with a cancer diagnosis there are plenty of reasons why you might be showing depressive signs.

There is a long history of doctors being dismissive of symptoms around the menopause, but luckily that is changing, and there is more information out there for perimenopausal women than there used to be. Having said that, this is still an area where you will need to stand your ground and insist on further support if you need it. I mentioned symptoms at about five oncologist appointments before it was suggested I could be referred to the menopause clinic.

If you would like to be able to have a baby after cancer treatment, there are several options available, including IVF, egg freezing and a newer technique known as ovarian tissue cryopreservation, which involves freezing some of your ovarian tissue before treatment begins. There are also hormone-blocking injections, such as Zoladex, that you can have during chemo to protect your ovaries. Sadly, none of these options comes with a cast-iron guarantee that you'll be able to conceive, but talk to your oncologist about the best decision for you. The loss of fertility can be incredibly upsetting, even if you already have a family or did not intend to have children, because it's that element of choice being taken away.

Hormone replacement therapy

The abrupt change can mean symptoms are more severe than they would be with natural menopause, which happens more gradually over a period of years. This can be a particularly challenging time because women who have had breast cancer are generally advised against taking hormone replacement therapy (HRT). It appears more clear-cut that women with hormone receptor positive breast cancer shouldn't have HRT, but even those of us who have been through treatment for HER2 or triple negative breast cancer are often advised against it. My oncologist said that HRT was not an option for me, because 'if it comes back, it might be the other type.'

Dani Binnington is a yoga teacher and host of the Menopause and Cancer podcast. She was diagnosed with breast cancer aged 33 and, after testing positive for the mutated BRCA1 gene, had her ovaries surgically removed to reduce her risk of ovarian cancer. Soon afterwards, her emotional wellbeing hit an all-time low with spiralling anxiety and fear of recurrence controlling her life. It took time, and everything from counselling and hypnotherapy to mindfulness and yoga (which she liked so much that she trained to be a yoga teacher), but eventually she got her life back on track.

She explains that the advice about women not having HRT after breast cancer treatment is based on two studies from Sweden – the HABITS study and the Stockholm study. These are the only randomised controlled trials that there have been.

We certainly need more information to make better-informed decisions. But most of us who have been through cancer treatment want to erase every element of risk that we possibly can, no matter how small. 'Our focus is on survival,' says Dani. 'If you're doing everything you can to reduce your risk of recurrence, then you won't want to have HRT initially, but, a few years down the line, maybe you can have that conversation.' Having said that, she has worked with women whose menopausal symptoms have been so severe that their marriage has broken up and they're feeling that they just can't go on like this. For these women, the evidence around risk of recurrence on HRT is not necessarily strong enough when weighed against the impact on their quality of life.

However, it's important to understand that HRT is not a miracle cure for symptoms, and many women struggle with it. So, as breast cancer patients, we shouldn't feel that our lives would automatically be so much better if only we could take HRT, as that may very well not be the case.

Symptoms

Symptoms of the menopause are so varied and wide-ranging that it can be difficult to identify them. Hot flushes and night sweats are the most obvious ones, but it also causes a grim catalogue of other symptoms including fatigue, insomnia, loss of libido, vaginal dryness, painful sex, dry eyes, dry skin, joint pains, muscle aches, bone thinning, headaches, poor memory and concentration (known as brain fog), irritability, anxiety, low mood, mood swings, lack of motivation, tearfulness, loss of joy and loss of confidence.

The symptoms can sometimes make themselves known in

bizarre ways, such as affecting my eyesight (which I mentioned in the chapter about chemo), and it also affected my driving in a way that made me feel as though I was going mad. Having been a relaxed and confident driver for years, I suddenly started panicking on the road, second guessing myself and not trusting my decisions when it came to changing lanes on the motorway or pulling out at a busy roundabout. I didn't connect this to the menopause until I attended one of Dani's workshops for breast cancer patients at Future Dreams House and realised other women were experiencing the same thing.

'These symptoms are like adding insult to injury,' says Dani – the injury clearly being the cancer. 'And it just feels like insult, after insult, after insult.'

As you may have noticed, lots of the above symptoms are similar to signs of depression, which has led to the often-quoted statistic that one in four women who go to the doctor with these symptoms are prescribed antidepressants, when they ought to be prescribed HRT. For us, with HRT generally off the medical menu, antidepressants can be a solution in some instances. Everyone is different, and a drug that works for one person may not work for another, but if you're struggling with symptoms please do talk to your doctor. I would suggest talking to your surgeon or oncologist in the first instance, rather than your GP, because they will have your cancer diagnosis at the forefront of their minds, and may be able to refer or prescribe you relevant support more quickly. In some cases, they may suggest it's simpler for you to speak to your GP about, for example, a prescription for antidepressants.

Another thing you might have noticed about the symptoms is that many of them are also side effects of chemotherapy, so segueing from being a chemo patient to a postmenopausal woman can be an extremely scary time, because you can feel as though something has been taken from you, and you can't get it back. Don't feel shy or embarrassed to talk about how you're feeling. There is clear evidence that falling off the oestrogen cliff can cause immense emotional upheaval, and it's perfectly natural for you to be finding this a confusing and distressing time.

The conversation around menopause is now very different compared to only a few years ago. There is a much more open dialogue, and many books, podcasts and TV series have sprung up about coping with peri- and postmenopausal life. However, so much of the focus of menopause discourse is about HRT, so it can make women who have been through (or are at high risk of) breast cancer feel excluded from the conversation.

'My research has shown that 92 per cent of women going through menopause after breast cancer feel isolated in their experience,' says Dani. 'It's a lonely and confusing place.' This is why she has worked to create a community of women going through the same thing, with her podcast, workshops and her Facebook group, which you can find by searching Menopause and Cancer Chat Hub.

'It's frustrating that there is such a focus on HRT as a solution, because there is so much that you can do outside of that,' says Dani. As with so many elements of cancer treatment, it is up to us to be as active as possible in our own recovery.

Bone health

Looking after your bones is so important after menopause, particularly for those of us who can't have HRT as that has a protective effect. Chemotherapy brought on early menopause for me, aged 40, which is common. Your menopause might be temporary or permanent, but it's more likely to be permanent if you are over 40. Your doctor might be able to suggest what will happen in your situation, but they are unlikely to be able to know for sure. In my case, it took several months of watching and waiting, then blood tests to check hormone levels several months apart, before it was agreed that I was postmenopausal. Only then did they do a bone density scan, which showed I had osteoporosis in my lower spine.

If your oncologist doesn't suggest a bone density test, it's worth requesting one. Also known as a DEXA scan, it's a quick and painless X-ray that can accurately show your risk of osteoporosis, or osteopenia, which is when you have lower bone density than average for your age but not low enough to be classed as osteoporosis. Either way, there is plenty that you can do to improve bone strength.

You may be prescribed a selective oestrogen receptor modulator called raloxifene, which has a similar effect to oestrogen on the bones, or a bisphosphonate such as zoledronic acid, generally known by the brand name Zometa. But there is much you can do to support bone health outside medication.

Movement is vital, because your bones are living tissue, and they get stronger when you use them. That's why keeping up with exercise as you age is so important for everyone, but particularly if you've been through cancer treatment.

Weight-bearing exercise – meaning everything from skipping and squats to actually lifting weights – is one of the best things you can do for strengthening both muscles and bones. Why do muscles matter in this context? Well, as your muscles get stronger, they pull harder, meaning your bones are more likely to become stronger, too. Gradually increasing the weight of what you lift is known as progressive resistance training, and research studies have shown that this is likely to be the best type of muscle-strengthening exercise for bone strength.

Calcium supplements are generally only needed if recommended by a doctor, as too much calcium can increase your risk of other health problems, and most people should be able to get enough from food. Cow's milk, yoghurt and cheese are great sources so, if you're dairy intolerant, make sure you're eating things like almonds, sesame seeds, broccoli and green leafy vegetables. But not spinach because that contains oxalate, which means the calcium isn't released into your bones. (Spinach is great in lots of ways, but not for calcium.) Lots of dairy-free milks, such as almond, soy or oat milk, are also fortified with calcium. However, you'll need to buy the non-organic version because the rules for organic produce prevent them from being fortified with vitamins and minerals.

Get adequate vitamin D – it's necessary for the body to absorb calcium. This means getting outside in the warmer months and supplementing when there is less sun in the sky.

Smoking slows down the cells that build bone in your body, so if you smoke then maybe looking after your bone health could be the extra incentive you need to stop for good.

Alcohol. If you drink, it's worth cutting down for many reasons, but specifically the Royal Osteoporosis Society says: 'If you drink a lot of alcohol, your risk of osteoporosis and broken bones is significantly higher.' This is because the liver plays an important part in bone metabolism. Alcohol has also been known to trigger hot flushes.

Hydration is vital for bone health. A lack of water to transport minerals and allow cells to function properly can lead to bone loss. And, since water also helps clear the body of toxins, dehydration can cause a build-up in the bones, leading to inflammation and a breakdown in bone mass.

All of this advice for bone health is good advice for menopause-related symptoms and general wellbeing, so it's worth following, even if you're getting regular Zometa infusions.

Your brain

Drinking plenty of water also supports brain function, and there has been research showing that being even slightly dehydrated can exacerbate brain fog and irritability.

Some people swear by supplements, such as Brain Select, which can help if you're lacking certain nutrients in your diet. Brain Select is largely a B-vitamin complex, so can be helpful if you don't eat meat, fish, eggs or dairy. If you're already taking a multivitamin, do check that you're not over-supplementing, as mega-dosing on vitamins has been debunked as a helpful thing to do and can sometimes even be harmful.

This is one area where starting a regular practice to relax and clear your mind can be enormously helpful in your brain's recovery and brain cell regeneration. This might include things you can do yourself such as breathwork or meditation. There are plenty of YouTube videos, and apps such as Calm, for this, but it can be as simple as sitting and focusing on your breath for a few minutes. One 70-something woman who had breast cancer at my age, and contacted me on Instagram, told me that Transcendental Meditation had changed her life, and made her brain sharper than it had been in years.

There are also therapies that have been shown to calm your mind, including massage, reflexology and reiki. Finding a great therapist is key, so ask around, engage with local breast cancer groups, and accept that it might take a bit of trial and error to find what's right for you. These treatments can quickly start to become expensive; if you're struggling, look into what's available within the NHS. Earlier, I mentioned the distance reiki that I had during my chemotherapy. It was arranged by the NHS and, had it not been for the pandemic, that would have taken place in person. So do talk to your breast care nurse about what complementary therapies might be available to you.

Your vagina

I know, talking about your vagina to a man in an NHS lanyard is pretty high on most people's awkwardometer. Assuming you're already doing your pelvic floor exercises (there are several apps you can download to remind you, including a good NHS one called Squeezy), there is plenty more you can do to support your vaginal health. It's embarrassing to raise vaginal issues with your doctor. So credit to Professor Peter Schmid, who brought up vaginal dryness in our conversation before I had to mention it. He also conceded that there are many medical professionals who find it hard to talk about – which doesn't help us, as patients. Vaginal dryness is an extremely common symptom of the menopause, and can be so severe that women are unable to do activities like ride a bike, or sit comfortably on a stool, never mind have sex. Then there is the fact that sexual problems are often exacerbated by psychological issues after cancer treatment, when many of us have a body that has been through the wringer and often looks quite different. Psychosexual counselling can be a huge support in that area, and there are also practical steps you can take to improve conditions in your vagina.

First of all, you need to start taking care of your vagina in the same way that you probably already do with your face: by keeping it well moisturised. Unfortunately, there are lots of products out there that advertise themselves as being for vaginal dryness but which are so full of perfumes and chemicals that they can actually make the situation worse. The ones that come highly recommended by experts are two brands: Yes and Sylk. Yes can actually be prescribed on the NHS, so you can ask for it specifically. Both brands make vaginal moisturisers, which can be used regularly for improving hydration, and vaginal lubricants that are specifically for making sex more comfortable. There are water-based and oil-based options for lubricants, with the main difference being that oil-based lubricants last longer, so don't have to be reapplied during sex, but they don't actually hydrate the skin in the way that water-based lubricants do, so many people choose to use them together.

There are also now brands of locally applied HRT, which come either in the form of a cream to apply directly to your vagina, or a pessary that you pop right up there. It's effective for the treatment of vaginal symptoms such as dryness, soreness, itching, burning and uncomfortable sex caused by oestrogen deficiency. And, since it doesn't enter your blood stream, it's considered safe for women who are advised against HRT. Most women can actually now buy it over the counter in the UK, but – not if you've had breast cancer! So ask your doctor about getting it on prescription.

I highly recommend episode 12 of Dani's podcast, Menopause and Cancer, which is an interview with menopause specialist and GP Dr Charlotte Gooding and Samantha Evans, co-founder of sex-toy company Jo Divine. It's packed with really practical advice and, if you haven't heard the words 'vaginal dryness' enough here, there's plenty more where that came from.

Herbal remedies

You may hear women raving about certain herbal remedies, saying that black cohosh or St John's wort has changed their life. But you will also hear just as many women say that they tried them and found zero benefit. This is because everyone reacts to things differently and, if you are going to try a herbal remedy, please don't just go to your local health store and buy a tub of St John's wort for £5.99. There is every chance that it'll be full of bulking agents and fillers, plus some herbal supplements even interfere with prescribed medication, so definitely don't start on them without checking that first. The only way to approach herbal remedies is to have a consultation with an accredited herbal specialist, for a personalised prescription. If you want to try that, you can find one on the website of the National Institute of Medical Herbalists.

Conventional drugs

Many women who have been through cancer treatment have an intense aversion to any further medication, and understandably want to avoid as many drugs as possible. Partly because they might still be reeling from the brutal side effects of chemotherapy or other treatments, and partly because they have started to feel like a human medical waste disposal unit. That's certainly how I felt after treatment. I didn't want to put anything pharmaceutical into my body unless absolutely necessary. For others, however, certain medications can be life-changing. I am clearly not a doctor and, even if I were, I wouldn't be able to make sweeping recommendations about drugs, as everyone is different and reacts to medication in a slightly different way.

Having said that, there are several non-hormonal treatments that have been mentioned by Dani and other menopause experts that I avidly follow, such as Annice Mukherjee. I'll list a few non-hormonal (and therefore safe for breast cancer) treatments here – with the caveat again that I am not recommending anything in particular – so that you can do your own research on them and discuss with your doctor.

- Clonidine can help reduce hot flushes and night sweats, as well as migraines.
- Citalopram and sertraline are both a type of antidepressant called selective serotonin reuptake inhibitor (SSRI). They can be prescribed for low mood, anxiety and panic attacks.
- Mirtazapine is an antidepressant that can make you very drowsy, so can be effective if you're struggling with insomnia, as well as low mood.

- Ovestin is a non-hormonal treatment that has an oestrogen-like effect on the vagina, counteracting vaginal dryness.
- Melatonin is a prescription-only medication that can improve sleep. It's available over the counter in the US.

Dani's advice when it comes to medication is to find your own way, and not be overly led by what others are doing. 'This is your life,' she says, 'so do your research, listen to your body and find what works for you.'

A positive change?

Once you've found what works for you, this could be the start of a brilliant new chapter in your life. While this can be a difficult time for many women, and it's important to talk about the symptoms so that we can address them, I wholeheartedly encourage you to try not to focus on all the doom and gloom. As Kristin Scott Thomas's character says in season two of *Fleabag,* the menopause is 'horrendous ... but then it's magnificent'.

In China, the menopause is known as the Second Spring. It's seen as a new beginning, where women are free from the pain and disruption of periods and childbirth. They have more confidence, wisdom and experience - and they're respected for that. It's a far cry from British work culture, which has seen anxiety-wracked midlife women trying to cool down in office toilet cubicles, lest anyone knows they're having a hot flush. Happily, this is changing. More slowly than it should but it is changing.

So please don't feel as though these unpleasant symptoms

are something that you just have to live with. And don't let any doctor fob you off by saying it's 'just the menopause'. Yes, it's a common experience, but that doesn't mean we're not entitled to the tools that can help us through it. Dani compares it to age-related macular degeneration. 'It would be like saying of people who were struggling with their eyesight: "Reading glasses exist, but we're not going to tell you about them." It's madness.'

I recommend a book by endocrinologist Dr Annice Mukherjee called *The Complete Guide to the Menopause*. It's one of the most practical handbooks I've come across – perfect for you if you wish this chapter were a whole book written by a hormone specialist. Dr Mukherjee has been through her own breast cancer diagnosis so, unlike many books about the menopause, it's not fixated on HRT as a solution.

Dr Mukherjee is a big advocate of movement as a way to deal with many symptoms, particularly after cancer treatment. 'It works through metabolic effects,' she explains, 'for stress reduction, improving sleep, body composition, glucose metabolism, cardiovascular health and much more. Regular exercise also reduces breast cancer recurrence by up to 55 per cent. If exercise was a drug, it would be the best on the market.' She has gone as far as to say, 'Exercise is my HRT.' If that won't get you moving, I don't know what will.

Dani Binnington reiterates this, adding that movement with a calming element like yoga can be good for stress levels. She also recommends complementary therapies like acupuncture and mindfulness for managing symptoms. 'We have studies proving that these things work,' she says. 'People often want to just take a pill and have their symptoms fixed but, if you put in the effort, it really does pay off.' So that means making time for exercise, getting enough quality sleep, managing stress and eating well (specifically, a wide range of plant foods and enough protein).

And do track your symptoms, because it *is* possible to have better care on the NHS. The services are there if you know to ask for them. Knowledge is power, and knowing what to ask the doctor for is the first step towards feeling better. As Dani says: 'You deserve to feel well.' And it's quite heartbreaking that so many of us have to be reminded of that.

Coping with the menopause without HRT

Karen Newby, a nutritionist with a BSc in nutritional medicine, and the author of *The Natural Menopause Method*, shares her top five tips.

1. Love your liver

Your liver has been through a lot with treatment and it's vital for detoxifying excess hormones. We can support this major multitasking organ through gentle liver tonics such as hot water with lemon in the morning, reducing stressors like caffeine and alcohol, and increasing consumption of cruciferous vegetables such as cabbage, cauliflower, radishes, broccoli and brussels sprouts, which help the liver work more efficiently.

2. Love your gut

Our gut is the biggest defence against the outside world, aside from the skin. It's home to two-thirds of our immune system, and it's also where we make most of our serotonin, the happiness neurotransmitter. Increase plant-based fibre slowly to help the bacteria that eat it gradually multiply, avoiding bloating or gas. Your gut loves fermented foods, Jerusalem artichokes, asparagus, leeks and all brightly coloured fruits and vegetables, which help repair the gut lining.

3. Beat hot flushes

Try keeping a hot flush diary to identify your triggers. Common ones are:

- Stimulants such as caffeine, sugar and alcohol.
- Stress. Try deep breathing if you feel a flush coming on.

Phytoestrogens can mimic oestrogen in a way that is not harmful and can reduce symptoms. Try tofu, miso, ground linseed, nuts, fennel, parsley, beans, lentils, chickpeas and green vegetables. Cooling foods include apples, pears, lemon, cucumber and celery.

4. Balance your blood sugar

Blood sugar rollercoasters increase stress hormones and exacerbate symptoms like hot flushes, irritability, anxiety and low mood. They can also deplete essential nutrients needed for energy, such as B vitamins. Sugary foods and refined carbs are like putting petrol on the fire: the flames burn super bright but don't last long, hence the blood sugar low. Whereas protein is like putting coal on the fire: the flames don't burn as bright but they kick off more heat and last for longer, giving you a drip feed of energy.

5. Rest and repair

Sleep is crucial for the body to repair itself. Magnesium is known as nature's tranquilliser, and you can absorb it through Epsom salts in a bath. Don't eat too late, as the heat from digestion can keep us awake. Alcohol massively affects restorative sleep and can also make us feel anxious the next day. It requires zinc to detox it from the body – and zinc is one of our anti-anxiety minerals. If you wake up in the night, try a breathing exercise to put your body back in rest and digest mode. And keep your phone outside the bedroom!

Secondary Breast Cancer

People often talk about breast cancer as being one of the most treatable and curable cancers there is, but this is of little comfort to the 11,500 women in the UK who die of secondary (also known as metastatic) breast cancer every year.

This is the section that I felt least comfortable writing. After treatment for primary breast cancer, fear of recurrence is so real and visceral, you might find (like I did) that you need to step back from reading or hearing about cases where the cancer has returned and spread to other parts of the body. However, as a result of the fact that most people with a breast cancer diagnosis are able to have curative treatment, women with secondary breast cancer can feel forgotten or ignored, so it's really important to address.

First, let's clarify the terminology. Breast cancer recurrence *can* be treatable, particularly if it's a local recurrence, i.e. it comes back in the breast, chest or armpit area. Locally advanced breast cancer, or regional recurrence, means the cancer has spread to the chest wall or the lymph nodes around the chest, neck or under the breast bone.

Secondary, or metastatic breast cancer, has spread through the lymphatic or blood system to other parts of the body, usually the bones, lungs, liver or brain. Even though the cancer is no longer focused in the breast, this is still considered breast cancer, and is quite distinct from a separate diagnosis of, for example, lung cancer.

Once this spread has happened, there is treatment available to manage the growth of the cancer, but it usually can no longer be cured. The exception to this is if the metastases (or mets, as they're known) are small and few, then this is known as oligometastatic breast cancer (OMBC), and there is a chance that it can be treated with curative intent. Patients with OMBC have talked about feeling as though they are in a kind of limbo between primary and secondary breast cancer, but it's becoming better understood by the medical community.

Again, I want to reassure you with the reminder that breast cancer recurrence rates are low. We know this from looking at the number of patients diagnosed, and comparing that with the mortality rate for breast cancer. However, there are no official statistics on the number of people living with a secondary diagnosis.

Professor Carlo Palmieri is consultant in medical oncology at the Clatterbridge Cancer Centre in Liverpool. In 2022, he used hospital episode statistics to estimate the number of people living with metastatic breast cancer in England, and how this figure had changed over the previous five years. His research shows that in 2020/21 there were 57,215 patients living with metastatic breast cancer. These numbers had increased steadily over the previous five years, rising from 38,350 in 2016/17. 'This is the first time that the number of people living with metastatic breast cancer in England has been estimated,' says Professor Palmieri. 'Previous estimations that 35,000 individuals are living with it in the UK are an underestimation, as we have calculated there are over 57,000 such people in England alone.'

'Secondary breast cancer is an invisible disease,' says Laura Price, journalist and author of the brilliant *Single Bald Female,* a cancer-inspired novel. 'With primary cancers, we are used to seeing people with bald heads, being on chemo and talking about finishing treatment, but secondary cancer is much more nuanced. It's something you die from, but it's also something you live with – emphasis on *live* – and people can live quite normal lives, continuing to do their jobs and go on holiday.' Depending on the type and grade of the cancer, you can live well for years in many cases, and it's getting better all of the time thanks to scientific advances.

Laura was initially diagnosed with ER+ breast cancer when she was 29. She had wide local excision surgery followed by chemo and radiotherapy. Ten years later, in 2022, she experienced chest pains and then learned that the cancer had spread to her sternum bone and was now incurable. She presently takes Zoladex, letrozole and ribociclib, and has had surgery to remove her sternum bone. 'Like with mental illness, you can't necessarily "see" secondary breast cancer when you look at someone, yet that person may be suffering side effects such as extreme fatigue,' she says. 'That's why it's so important for us to practise kindness at all times. You never know what someone is going through so, whether you're in the workplace or on the Tube, try to be considerate and understanding.'

The amount of time that a person can live after a secondary breast cancer diagnosis varies wildly, and is dependent on many different factors, so I'm not going go into numbers of years because, as Laura says, life is (or should be) about quality rather than quantity. As one woman living with secondary breast cancer explained it to me: 'It's about the life in your years, rather than the years in your life.'

Laura remembers the day she was diagnosed, and had to tell her partner the devastating news. 'I said to him: "Life is going to be so much more beautiful for us now. We're going to make so much of every single moment we have together, whether my life is long or short." I'm not going to say that cancer is a gift but, when you know you will die much sooner than you had hoped, it allows you to decide what you want to do with that time,' she explains. 'Focus on what you want to do with your life, and do it now, instead of putting it off for some distant day that may never come.'

Jo Taylor founded the online platform ABCDiagnosis after being diagnosed with primary breast cancer aged 38. She realised that reconstructive surgery options were not the same for women all around the UK, where it can be something of a postcode lottery. She was determined, did her own research and requested a second opinion, ultimately finding a surgeon that she was happy with. But she knew that many women don't advocate for themselves in the same way, and wanted to create a resource where they could see all of their options easily. 'I wanted the patient's voice to come through,' she says, 'as the information from specialists often takes the form of: "Here's a leaflet, read it." I feel that everyone should be empowered with as much knowledge as possible.'

Seven years later, she was diagnosed with secondary breast cancer and, again, felt disheartened with the lack of information coming from medical professionals – many of whom don't even tell patients what to look out for in terms of recurrence. 'Sadly oncologists, surgeons and even breast care nurses have this mentality of "it's too scary", but awareness is so important,' she says. 'It's great that everyone knows about checking their breasts, but it's also important that people know the red flag signs of secondary breast cancer. I've even been told not to use the phrase "red flag" as it scares people.'

So she created an infographic showing the signs of breast cancer recurrence, which you can see at ABCDiagnosis.co.uk. NHS England signposts to it and the NHS in Greater Manchester now includes it in their end-of-treatment summary reports. Jo has had feedback that people wouldn't have received their diagnosis so quickly without it.

THE MAIN SYMPTOMS OF RECURRENCE INCLUDE:

- BRAIN: Frequent headaches, vomiting in the morning, dizziness, visual disturbance, seizure, impaired intellectual function, mood swings, balance issues and fatigue.
- BONES: Pain with no obvious cause or trauma, most commonly in the thigh, arm, ribs or back. It can be a dull ache or a sharp shooting pain.
- LUNGS: Sharp pain on breathing, in chest and back, as well as a non-productive cough.
- LYMPH NODES: Swelling or lumps and pressure in the chest, underarm or neck.
- LIVER: Bloating, affected appetite, weight loss, fatigue, and pain on right-hand side.

One of the reasons that it's so important to be aware of the signs is because you won't be offered routine scans unless you have worrying symptoms. If you do, you can call your breast nurse and be seen in the breast clinic very quickly, so always be aware that this is an option. In terms of scans, patients (in England and Wales, at least) are offered mammograms (on the remaining breast if you've had a mastectomy), even though recurrence is unlikely to occur in the other breast.

Partly to try and make sense of this bewildering state of affairs, Jo founded MET UP UK, with the aim of advocating for women with metastatic breast cancer. 'We are advocates, campaigners and activists who demand change for awareness, drug access, clinical trials and data. We're not even counted when alive,' she adds, referring to official breast cancer statistics that don't differentiate between a primary and a secondary diagnosis, 'only when we're dead.'

MET UP UK runs a campaign called Darker Pink during Breast Cancer Awareness Month, highlighting the fact that many people with metastatic breast cancer can feel excluded from the conversation, as if they are some kind of lost cause. Jo's aim is for it to become a chronic disease that can be managed for a lifetime, rather than a death sentence. 'I'm one of the lucky ones, living well nine years later and still on first-line treatment which, in my case, is a Phesgo injection of Perjeta and Herceptin,' she says. 'So I am lucky – many of my friends are dead, as they ran out of treatment options – but I have had 14 surgeries in the last eight years, and who wants their sternum removed?'

If you have a primary breast cancer diagnosis, the purpose of this chapter is not to scare you. The vast majority of women diagnosed with breast cancer – 76 per cent – will get better, and survival rates are improving all the time. But it's important to talk about this so that you know what to look out for, and any recurrence can be diagnosed and treated as quickly as possible.

The Best Thing That Could Have Happened to You?

When I was diagnosed, a stranger messaged me on Instagram saying: 'You might not be ready to hear this yet, but breast cancer was the best thing that ever happened to me.' She was right: I absolutely was not ready to hear that at the time.

This reframing of the experience of breast cancer initially sounds completely mad, particularly when you're in the throes of treatment. But you'd be surprised by how possible, and even how common, it can be.

It's something that you are unlikely to get on board with until you have found your way through the anger about the injustice of your diagnosis, and the grief for your old life, and those 'why me?' moments lying awake in the early hours. But then many people feel that once they have managed to accept their cancer diagnosis, they can start to feel ready to acknowledge the positive things it has given them.

This turnaround might happen for several reasons. First of

all, anything that heightens your awareness of death makes you more capable of appreciating life: whether that be your friends, family, health or work. We feel this to some degree when we read a news story about a horrific event in which people have died. Friends and colleagues will talk in hushed tones about how the incident 'puts things in perspective', and it does for a while but, as everyday annoyances stack up, that perspective tends to disappear.

Having cancer provides this perspective on a longer-term basis, and many people make a big life change after a diagnosis. They might quit their job or leave a bad relationship. They might start saying 'no' to things they don't want to do but previously felt they should, while saying 'yes' to things they want but have not felt brave enough to do.

When you learn to embrace the briefness of life, you start to recognise more moments as being special. Because human life *is* brief compared to, say, an oak tree. And that's true for all of us, although those of us with a cancer diagnosis are more keenly aware of it.

If you want a lesson in making the most of the time that we have on this earth, then talk to someone with secondary breast cancer and you'll soon be looking at life with a renewed sense of gratitude. This can shape how you feel about everything. For example, you might no longer say: 'I have to go to work today', because really it's: 'I *get* to go to work today'.

This reframing can be powerful, but it won't happen without some effort on your part. As we know, our brains are designed to focus on the negative, and anticipate the worst-case scenario. Hope is a conscious choice that you have to make, despite all evidence to the contrary. You have to *choose* to focus on hope rather than fear.

And part of this is about learning to accept uncertainty. I get so many messages on social media from people struggling to cope with their own diagnosis, or that of someone they love, reaching out to me for advice. Sadly, I can't tell them what they really want to hear, which is: 'Everything's going to be fine.' Nobody can ever tell us that. But then, cancer or no cancer, none of us truly knows what the future holds, and all we can do is find ways to live as well as we can, while we can.

Harvard psychologist Dan Gilbert wrote the 2006 book, *Stumbling on Happiness*. He says that we have a 'psychological immune system', giving us a remarkable ability to not only survive but thrive in the face of adversity. The trouble is, he says, we often underestimate it. This concept is called 'immune neglect', and it can mean that people stay for too long in relationships that are not working or jobs they hate, because they underestimate how well they'll be able to cope with getting a divorce or losing their regular salary.

For his research, he spoke to people who have been through horrific experiences, such as losing a child. 'They never say: "I'm glad that happened,"' he explains. 'But if you ask them to name the good and the bad things that have come from it, they tend to name more good than bad.' That, to me, is astonishing.

This isn't to diminish trauma or to tell you to simply pull yourself together, but his research should give you a sense of optimism about what you may be capable of in the future. As he says: 'If you understand the power of the psychological immune system, our remarkable ability to rationalise in the face of adversity, it makes you braver.'

You are dealing with something that nobody would ever have chosen. If you can get through this, then you can do anything.

Karen Verrill, centre head at Maggie's Newcastle, tells me that reaching this mindset may not be easy, but it is possible, and there is lots of support out there to help you. 'At Maggie's we have psychologists who will do one-to-ones and provide people with coping strategies to process everything and work through it,' she says. 'We also have a mindfulness course, one on stress management, living with uncertainty, and the Where Now? course (*see page 187*). It's so important because if you can feel good in your head, then you tend to feel good in your body.'

The problem is encouraging people to take those steps for their mental wellbeing, particularly when it's easy to be cynical about such things. 'I'm not saying "be positive, be brave, you're inspirational", and all those things that people say because they mean well but can be quite annoying to hear,' says Karen. 'It's about prioritising yourself, which women find hard because they feel guilty. They never think that they've done enough. Anything that goes wrong, women put it on themselves. They spend so much time worrying about what they *should* be doing, rather than thinking about what they *want* to do.'

Karen says the first step is acknowledging how you feel, rather than pretending to be fine in order to protect those around you. 'Following treatment for breast cancer, I call the next phase the "recovery period",' she says. 'It's a time to get yourself back into a better place in the world. If you want to improve your general wellbeing, that starts with your mental wellbeing. You have to start a new mindset, and think of yourself, instead of everybody else, first.'

Taking a pause

I love this idea of a recovery period. It's like the word 'convalescence', which makes me think of fragile eighteenth-century waifs, travelling to a spa town to 'take the waters' and heal. In the nineteenth century, Florence Nightingale recommended building convalescent cottages in the country or by the sea. The fact that we lack a modern equivalent is admittedly because we have vastly improved medicine, housing and sanitation, but it also shows what little value we place on the concept of recovery. Do not be afraid to lean in to this now.

This is the time to take care of yourself. Don't overcommit to work, family or social events, if you can avoid it. Eat well, go on long walks, drink lots of water, go to bed early. Small, manageable steps are key, because this transition is tough.

You've probably become accustomed to things happening quickly. From a meal arriving at the tap of a screen, to a work negotiation coming to fruition thanks to a diplomatic Zoom call. Everything is so instant, we no longer know how to be patient, and it can be frustrating to realise that one of the most important elements of rebuilding your life after breast cancer is time.

One psychotherapist I spoke to described how, in the period after cancer treatment, we try to fight against the trauma of what we've been through, and push away the fear and anxiety about recurrence. But you can't push them away, because if you do they will only get bigger. Instead, accept anything that comes up, try to process it, and be assured that it will get better with time. I'm sorry not to have better news on this point, but you have to feel all of those bleak feelings. You have to welcome them in, acknowledge how horrible it feels, but know that this is normal.

And - here's the tricky bit - once you've acknowledged them, you have to release them. As the saying goes: let your feelings in but don't make them tea. Use every tool and technique that appeals to try and let them go. Get therapy. Do yoga. Try energy healing. Learn to meditate. I'm not saying do *all* of these things, but experiment to find what works for you.

Your challenge now is to become the most Zen version of yourself. One way or another, you'll get through the next couple of years - and you do need to allow at least a year for this process, because we're not talking about a few weeks here. Accepting that this is your reality right now is hard, but it can help to realise that you won't feel this way for ever.

In the meantime, you might find it helpful to have a break from social media. I have talked a lot about the benefits of social media in this book. The breast cancer community on Instagram was of enormous support to me during my treatment and beyond. But even I have to step back sometimes. It can be something as simple as seeing an image that reminds you of your pre-cancer life. Or, if you now follow lots of breast cancer accounts (as I do), then you will inevitably sometimes see bad news, which can bring your fear and anxiety bubbling back to the surface.

Seeking positive stories

A perfect illustration of how social media can be both a blessing and a curse is a quick glance at my direct messages. For every heartbreaking DM from somebody with a new diagnosis who is feeling distraught and desperate for reassurance, there is a supportive message from someone keen to tell me what they've found has helped them through it. My favourite messages are the ones from women in their 70s and older, who tell me about their own cancer diagnosis when they were around my age, and how well they are doing now. I love that these women take the time to tell me their stories, since they know how I'm feeling, and how important it is to hear what life could be like many years on. It makes me realise that, once you're in this club, you're in it for good. And that's not necessarily a bad thing if you're able to role model a happy, healthy cancer-free life for anyone newly diagnosed. I know that every cancer is different and you shouldn't compare your own diagnosis to someone else's, but these messages mean so much to me because they help me focus on a positive outcome, making it easier to choose hope. Here are some of my favourites:

Mary: 'Today is 25 years since I was diagnosed with aggressive breast cancer, and most recent scan results are clear. I remember hoping to live until my youngest went to secondary school [she was seven]. Now, I have two gorgeous grandsons.'

Dolores: 'Go girl! I did the journey myself in 1994 and 1997, very aggressive stage three cancers. I am still here, and I believe you will be here in 28 years (and longer) too.'

Susan: 'Don't listen to the statistics – they told me I was at high risk of recurrence and I was scared for a long time until I realised that is no way to live your life. I am now nearly 30 years on from my diagnosis. Focus on hope!'

It can really help to identify positive role models. Happily, this is much easier now than it used to be, as there is now far greater awareness about breast cancer. Activist Gloria Steinem has talked about how she 'didn't know how to enter the last third of life' after being diagnosed with breast cancer back in

1986, because 'there were so few role models. I thought, this is how it's going to end. It was like falling off a cliff because I couldn't see enough people ahead of me.'[3]

So identify those role models. Personally, I enjoy reading about director Sam Taylor-Johnson living her best life in Los Angeles with her hot young husband, years after overcoming diagnoses for both breast and bowel cancer.

But also see friends in real life, rather than just liking their pictures, and surround yourself with positive people. It is said that you become the average of the five people that you spend most time with, so think about who they are. You can't necessarily change who you sit near to at work or at a family gathering, but you can change who you spend time with outside that. Identify the people that inspire you and bring you joy, and make an effort to see them more often. You might have heard of the drains and radiators analogy, as a way to differentiate the people who warm you up versus the ones that suck your energy away. What you have been through will almost certainly have brought those differences into sharp relief.

Designing Your Identity

I hope this book has galvanised you to work through and accept your most uncomfortable feelings, find ways to process your trauma, and make a conscious choice to look to the future with hope. Now, you are ready to rebuild yourself, from the ground up.

Cancer absolutely decimated my physical identity, from losing my hair and eyebrows during chemo, to feeling too weak to run alongside my son's bike, to a post-mastectomy body that is a daily reminder of what I've been through. But the destruction of my psychological identity has arguably been even more difficult to deal with, partly because it's less visible. One day, I was a thriving, energetic, healthy 40-year-old. Within a year, I was broken, after chemotherapy, surgery, radiotherapy and further adjuvant chemo.

But a year after *that,* you might assume I was getting back to my old self. My lashes and brows were back, and my hair had regrown sufficiently to have a short bob. On the outside, I looked normal. On the inside, however, I was struggling enormously with all-consuming fear of recurrence, as well as lymphoedema, osteoporosis, mood swings, brain fog and a litany of other menopause-related symptoms, including skin that seems to be ageing in dog years. All I wanted was to be my old self again.

It has been extremely hard to learn that I have to let go of the old version of myself and, to be honest, it's an ongoing process. But there is a lot I have found that can help.

In 2022, researchers Madeline Toubiana, Trish Ruebottom and Luciana Turchick Hakak presented the results of a decade spent studying how people react to drastic change. Over the course of hundreds of interviews, they identified a phenomenon they call 'identity paralysis' – a feeling of stuck-ness after a huge change in life (such as a cancer diagnosis) that left people feeling angry, frustrated and hopeless. Interestingly, this was the case even when the big change in a person's life was arguably a positive one, such as getting out of prison.

By interviewing people who were coping well with such transitions, they identified three positive strategies that we can all use. They are:

1. Acknowledge and process difficult emotions, which means talking them through rather than ignoring them (sorry to bang on about this, but the evidence is certainly stacking up as to how important it is).
2. Look for a story that you can tell about why the change turned out to be positive. For example, you might have a new appreciation of the small things in life, or you have instigated a healthy habit such as embracing exercise or drinking less alcohol.
3. Find something that symbolically marks the end of one identity and the birth of another. It can be a randomly chosen milestone, such as a birthday or new year, or a

physical symbol or ritual. I got a tattoo to mark the end of treatment: a triangle on my wedding-ring finger representing the mathematical symbol for change, and the Greek letter D – a tribute to the Dean family (specifically Jonathan) for getting me through. And you may remember in the chapter about chemo, I mentioned buying a big, cosy zip-up hoodie? Well, I wore it to every single scan, blood test and trip to the chemo ward. When treatment finished, donating that hoodie to the clothes bank felt symbolic of moving on. One psychotherapist I spoke to suggested a ritual where you write down all of your darkest fears about breast cancer, and then burn them, ideally during a full moon. I laughed when she told me this, but she said it can be extremely powerful in enabling your brain to move on. I tried it and admit that it felt cathartic. At the very least, it's a fun little bonfire.

Who do you want to be?

Identity change is never easy, but acknowledging that it is necessary and inevitable is the first step towards using this transition to design your new identity. Why is this so important? Well, the kind of person that you believe yourself to be subconsciously influences every decision that you make. Think of all the times that you have decided not to do something because of what kind of person you are:

'I'm no good with money.'
'I'm just not a sporty type.'
'I can't cook.'
'I'm not a morning person.'

You're more likely to be capable of giving up smoking if,

rather than saying, 'I'm trying not to smoke,' you say 'I'm a non-smoker.' If you're trying to instigate a habit of running, don't say, 'I'm trying to find time to run three times a week.' Just say: 'I'm a runner.'

Say it to yourself, and out loud to anyone who's interested. Write it in your social media bio. It's one thing to say, 'I'm the type of person who *wants* this,' but quite another to say, 'I'm the type of person who *is* this.'

We reconstruct ourselves several times over the course of our lives. It doesn't necessarily take a cancer diagnosis – it could be losing a job that was part of your identity, or going through a break-up, becoming a parent, losing someone you love, dealing with the menopause ... the list goes on. These moments cause self-reflection and personal re-evaluation. They change the shape of us, and force us to address what our values are, what gives our life purpose or meaning, and how we can use that information to rewrite the story of our life. That all sounds lovely, but the reality of it is hard. Like grief, it's something you have to push through. It's a cliché, but time is healing. Unfortunately, that also means it can't be rushed.

Identifying these moments that threaten your sense of self gives you the chance to seize control and rewrite the narrative, steering your identity towards who you want to be. I don't mean forcing yourself to be someone you're not, but rather working out what is important to you and living a more deliberate life. Your identity is not made of cement, it can be changed. Think of it as a sandcastle. You might spend years constructing it, but you can't control the tides and, inevitably, one day it'll get swept away. Rather than clinging to a castle that can't possibly last for ever, you can choose to enjoy the view of the beach, and the challenge of starting over with a totally new build.

I didn't want to accept the identity of being 'a cancer person', with the perceived associations of unsexy fragility. And the best way to reject one identity is to work out what you want your identity to be.

Clarifying your values

Your values are core beliefs, rather than something you value. For example, you might value a close friend, but the value attached to that is friendship. Here, I will list some common values. Read through the list and identify the ones that resonate most strongly with you, or you might come up with some of your own. Then go through your new list, comparing them with each other, until you are able to distil your values down to, say, five words that define who you want to be.

Creativity
Adventure
Pleasure
Simplicity
Family
Calm
Learning
Fun
Authenticity
Growth
Achievement
Spirituality
Toughness
Wealth

Altruism
Belonging
Challenge
Authority
Contribution
Independence
Courage
Empathy
Friendships
Generosity
Honesty
Boldness
Humour
Determination

Influence
Autonomy
Beauty
Integrity
Kindness
Leadership
Service
Recognition
Security
Longevity
Community
Love
Curiosity
Loyalty

Optimism	Stability	Strength
Peace	Wisdom	Joy
Compassion	Awareness	Gratitude
Purpose	Balance	Sustainability

Once you have your values, keep them at the forefront of your mind. You might have them on a Post-it note inside the front of your diary or notebook. You might stick them on your mirror, or have them saved in your phone. You could turn them into a mantra that you say to yourself every morning. The possibilities are endless, as long as you find a way to keep them in your mind.

A deeper sense of fulfilment is found when your values align with your actions. So remember the observation, usually attributed to Joan Baez, that 'action is the antidote to despair'.[4] And think of what you can do right now to move you towards where you'd prefer to be. You don't need to plan an exercise schedule or make some kind of overwhelming list. Just focus on the next thing – just one thing – and do that. And keep doing the next one thing

You are never too old to make this change. Whatever age you are now, your future self would love to be that. It's like the classic proverb (that I've seen attributed to both ancient China and the Stoics, and is now most commonly found in a cutesy font on Instagram), which says: 'The best time to plant a tree was 20 years ago; the next best time is today.' Because clearly, the best time to become who you want to be was 20 years ago, but the next best time is now.

The power of the mind

Now that you have identified what's important to you in terms of your values, you can define your intention. Everything in life starts with an intention. As a journalist, I've often been told to 'write the headline first', which means knowing what you want the piece to say before you start your research or interview anyone. Of course, if your research throws up an even more interesting headline, then you can change it. But it's useful to know where you're heading. What I'm encouraging you to do is write the headline of your life now.

Perhaps your intention is to travel the world, learn a language, write a book or celebrate your 50th wedding anniversary. It could turn out to be even better than you expected, but it's good to know where you want to be going, and believe that you can get there. To do this, you must let go of other people's opinions (and that pained sympathetic face they make whenever they ask how you're doing) and overcome that voice in your head. Have the strength to reject cynicism if it's no longer serving you.

There are neurological reasons why your beliefs about yourself actually change the direction in which your life goes. You will find people who swear by the magic of making a vision board or manifesting, but it isn't actually magic. According to neuroscientist and senior lecturer at MIT, Dr Tara Swart, focusing on an intention with tools such as visualisation actually works as a science. In her 2019 book, *The Source*, she explains how making a vision board of images of things that you want to manifest in your life actually primes your brain to take micro steps towards your goals every day. It works not by magic but by focusing your unconscious mind to zone in on what you have decided you want in life. And this is what keeping your values in mind can do, too.

PART IV:

FUTURE-PROOFING YOUR BODY

This section is all about the steps you can take to proactively reduce your risk of recurrence. It's never too early to start making positive lifestyle changes, so you can begin at any point on your journey. These steps can also help your body tolerate the onslaught of cancer treatment.

The first thing that I need to make clear is that I'm not here to make false promises or offer miracle solutions. Lifestyle factors certainly influence your risk of developing cancer; that's been proven. But there is also a lot that has not been proven, and there is so much about human biology that we have yet to understand.

We all know chain smokers who drink every day and live for a long time, and sadly many of us have known fit, healthy young people who have got cancer. Sometimes there really is no rhyme or reason to it. Yet, there is a huge amount of evidence that lifestyle can make a big difference in many cases.

The latest data by the World Cancer Research Fund (WCRF) found that, of the 387,000 people diagnosed with cancer in the UK between 2019 and 2020, 40 per cent of those cases (about 155,000) could have been avoided with lifestyle changes. This amounts to more than 400 people being diagnosed with preventable cancer every single day, in the UK. And that's an increase of 8,000 preventable cases compared with data from the previous two years. Again, the report clearly stated that not all cancers can be prevented, since there are many unmodifiable factors such as ageing and a family history of the disease. But it goes to show that there is a lot that people can do to help themselves live better, for longer.

The above statistics (and, let's face it, many statistics) have to be taken with a pinch of salt in terms of accuracy, because it's almost impossible to know with absolute certainty that a cancer was caused by lifestyle factors. So the actual figure may be higher or lower than reported.

'It's hard to put actual numbers on risk, and thus risk reduction, because anything you do (good or bad) is a relative change and not absolute,' says Dr Niamh Buckley of Queen's University Belfast. 'Breast cancer is so heterogeneous, so we have ideas of what the average risk is for any given group but, within that, there is going to be a lot of variability. It is very hard to measure how much you have reduced something when you didn't know what it was to start with.'

The other issue with talking about reducing your risk of recurrence is that people can start to worry that having cancer is somehow their fault. This is both wrong and heartbreaking. 'I hate seeing when people feel as though they're being blamed, like: "If you had lost a stone, you wouldn't have got cancer,"' says Dr Buckley. 'Obviously, yes, being as healthy as you can will help. But it's not necessarily always going to prevent something controlled by your genetic make-up. Sometimes biology is just too strong.'

I certainly never want anyone to feel 'blamed' for their cancer due to their lifestyle. Let's think about the word 'blame'. Do I think heavy smokers who get lung cancer are to blame for their disease? Absolutely not. A smoker is a person who has grown up in an environment where smoking is not only acceptable but often expected. They might experiment with smoking as a young person in order to fit in, then it becomes a habit, and a way of dealing with everything from stressful situations to social interactions. I wouldn't blame the smoker, I don't even blame so-called 'big tobacco'. There are many social and cultural factors that contribute to an environment that produces certain behaviours.

You don't have to look hard at the modern world to see that it encourages, or at least enables, a sedentary lifestyle fuelled by processed convenience foods and 'wine time'. I don't think 'blame' should play any part in it. The very concept of blame places all the onus on the individual, which is not helpful. But I also think that many health professionals are so cautious about not assigning blame that they let people down by not providing advice and support on the small, but potentially life-saving, steps that people can take to be healthier..

What I would like is for people to think of lifestyle choices in a different way. Not as a stick with which to beat yourself, or other people. But as an opportunity to seize the reins. Nobody wants to feel blamed. But most people like to feel empowered, with the responsibility to take control of their own health, without being overwhelmed by it.

And Dr Buckley agrees that making an effort to live well can only be beneficial. There are no drawbacks, after all. 'Everything and anything you can do to make you as healthy and as happy as you can be is a positive,' she says. 'It gives people something to focus on that is within their control.'

That sense of control is something that I was desperate for during cancer treatment, when so much feels so uncontrollable. I hated the feeling of not knowing why this had happened, and I asked many doctors why they thought I had developed breast cancer. I did have a family history, but the genetic testing came back clear. The best answer that any doctor could give me was that maybe I had a genetic mutation they had not yet discovered. More commonly they'd say it's 'just bad luck', which is hard to accept.

I personally feel (and maybe you do, too) that I'd be prepared to do anything and everything to increase my chances of never having to be back in that chemotherapy chair. So, even if the modifiable factor is small, that's enough for me to make a change.

Dr Liz O'Riordan is a breast surgeon who has had breast cancer, and has become known for dispelling breast cancer myths on social media with scientifically robust evidence-based take-downs. But, she tells me, there is convincing data that some things *can* reduce your risk of breast cancer. 'They're very simple and boring,' she warns, 'but the three things that we know can increase your risk are: not exercising, being overweight and binge-drinking alcohol. So tackling those has been proven to reduce the risk. But there's no guarantee it'll work because skinny, fit people can still get recurrence.'

There is much about biology that is not yet fully understood, but, interestingly, we don't necessarily have to simply accept the hand we are dealt when it comes to genetics. The ways in which our genes are activated or expressed can be altered by making healthier choices. 'It's called epigenetics, and part of my PhD was on this,' says Dr O'Riordan. 'It comes down to diet, sleep, exposure to chemicals, drinking and smoking. The more unhealthy your lifestyle is, your body is going to read your genes in a different way that may be more likely to cause problems in the future.'

This affects every process in your body, not just whether or not you get cancer, but it is certainly relevant in this context.

'Generally, cancer happens when there are spelling mistakes in the genes that either make a cell grow or stop it growing, and lifestyle may make you more likely to have those mistakes,' she explains, adding that healthy changes are always good, even if it sometimes feels as though the damage is already done.

If you're a parent, of course, you're in the privileged position of being able to intervene *before* the damage is done. 'If you've got children, you can help them live a healthier lifestyle, and you will reduce their chances of being ill in the future,' she says. 'That's a really powerful thing that people can do.'

Anyone who has kids knows that if you don't allow them to have sugar-packed foods occasionally, then they land face-first in the cake every time they go to a birthday party. The trick is to normalise healthy eating the majority of the time, and not make a big deal of it when you have the occasional ice cream. They do as you do, not as you say, and that's a good incentive. Not only for you to eat well, but also to move regularly, get enough sleep, take time to rest, wear sunscreen, don't smoke, have fun, fulfilling relationships, drink moderately, and basically model any behaviour that you would like your offspring to adopt for their long-term health and happiness.

Dr O'Riordan says it can be useful to think in terms of 80/20, i.e. if you're healthy 80 per cent of the time, then you can be pretty relaxed about what happens in the other 20 per cent. 'It's about having that balanced lifestyle,' she says, admitting that as a surgeon, she didn't always make the healthiest choices. 'When I got cancer, it was a wake-up call. I realised I need to look after myself. I need to exercise, I need to eat protein at every meal, and I need to say no to some stuff, because no one's going to do that for me.'

To me, this makes so much sense. In our polarised society,

where everything appears to be black or white, right or wrong, it's rare to find nuanced debate. It's even rarer to acknowledge that two seemingly opposing views can both be right, in their own way. I do believe that some cancers are going to occur no matter what you do. I also believe that lifestyle can have a huge impact on your risk of developing certain cancers and other diseases.

At the end of cancer treatment, I asked my oncologist if there were any day-to-day things I could do to reduce my risk of recurrence. 'It's the usual stuff,' she replied. 'Eat healthily and exercise.' She's right, of course, but the trouble is this advice is frustratingly vague. If you asked 10 different people to define a healthy diet, you could easily get 10 different answers. There are people who are passionate about being vegan, or gluten-free, or eating mostly raw food, or following a very low-carb diet like Keto, or fasting ... the list is seemingly endless. And I know that exercise is important, but is yoga enough or do I need to get really sweaty? And how often? I've heard strength training is important, not only for your bone health but also to reduce your risk of recurrence: does that mean I need to lift weights or does Pilates count?

What I want to do is cut through all the noise and provide clear, concise information that is genuinely helpful. Because the current advice is about as clear as a muddy puddle. I have spoken to experts to gather the best evidence-based information for simple lifestyle interventions that will have the biggest impact in terms of staying cancer-free.

And the great thing about these interventions is that they also reduce your risk of many other age-related conditions, including dementia, osteoporosis, diabetes and heart disease. 'Two-thirds of women diagnosed with primary breast cancer will die of old age,' says O'Riordan. 'They'll die of heart attacks and strokes. And eating healthily, exercising and sleeping well can reduce their risk of those things too, and delay that happening.'

You may well say that most people already know what they ought to be doing to improve their long-term health. But knowing it and doing it are two different things. A cancer diagnosis is horrible, yes, but it's also an opportunity to confront your own mortality and take matters into your own hands. People need a reason to actually do that, because it's human nature to scratch a current itch rather than think about long-term prevention. It's why we now see so many 'ticking time bomb' health issues that could have been avoided with some simple lifestyle interventions earlier on.

Tony Fadell, who invented the iPod, famously said that many more people buy painkillers than vitamins. It's not the best analogy considering the flourishing supplements market these days, but his point was: if you want to sell a product, focus on people's immediate pain-point, not some future improvement in their life. And the prevention of a far-off potential cancer diagnosis is not usually high on people's lists of immediate concerns. So think of ways in which these interventions can also make you happier in the short term, for example by improving your mental health and energy.

Make it doable

The other important thing with habit change is to make it small and achievable. Rather than throwing yourself into a hugely restrictive diet or punishing exercise regime, accept that piling pressure on yourself is counterproductive, and small steps are more effective in the long term – even if they don't feel as though they're doing much initially. As a starting point, think about four pillars: nutrition, movement, sleep and stress management. Which of those do you think needs a bit of attention in your life, and are there any simple, small steps that you can take to improve in this area? Remember, if you're going to stick with it, you need to make it easy and convenient. Get granular, and look at the architecture of your day:

- Could you fit in a 10-minute breathing practice before the rest of the household wakes up in the morning?
- Could you head into the bathroom five minutes earlier to do dry body brushing before your shower, to improve lymphatic flow?
- Could you do a 10-minute online yoga class straight after putting the kids to bed, before you settle down to watch Netflix?
- Could you turn a lunchtime run into a habit?

It can be easy to become obsessed with one area or another. Nutrition, for example, where people sometimes go crazy and cut out entire food groups. Or exercise: you don't have to go straight to training for a marathon. Consistent small actions are way more powerful than sweeping lifestyle changes that can be difficult to stick with.

The really brilliant thing about all this is that these choices affect those around you in a positive way. If you arrange to meet a friend for a walk instead of in the pub, that person has a healthier day. If you tell a colleague about how much yoga has helped you, they might take it up, too. If you start cooking from scratch more often at home, your whole household benefits. Once you start doing this, you'll realise that the ways in which you can pay it forward are endless.

Every cancer patient is an individual with their own distinct attitudes and ideas. You might be reading this feeling positive and energised and ready to focus your attention on all the ways that you can help your body to optimal health. Or you might be reading this feeling like lifestyle change is a slog that you can't face, particularly not at the same time as dealing with all the draining aspects of cancer treatment.

Mindset

If you're in any doubt as to why mindset is so important, two really interesting examples of research exist that illustrate it.

In one study, people were given a smoothie to drink. Half of them were told it was a nutrient-packed health drink, and the other half were told it was a sugary, McDonald's-style shake. The group that believed they were drinking something unhealthy thought it was far more delicious than the other group, even though it was exactly the same drink. And the results were not just based on what they said – the researchers actually tested their hormone levels and found that their biology showed they physiologically enjoyed the drink more when they thought it was less healthy. Their preconceptions about what something 'healthy' tastes like actually changed how much they enjoyed it.

Another study recruited cleaners, and told half of them that cleaning work is an excellent way to lose weight. Several weeks later, the cleaners in the group that expected to lose weight, had lost weight, while the other group hadn't.

The way that you approach something significantly affects your experience of it, so I want you to read this part of the book with an open mind, a willingness to try new things and an optimistic belief that it will do you good. You don't have to force yourself into a training regime that makes you miserable, or eat mushrooms if you hate them (side note: I hate mushrooms). But you do have to give things a go, in order to identify what works for you and what doesn't. You can choose to be an active participant in your own wellbeing rather than a passive victim.

Movement

You've no doubt noticed that the importance of physical activity has been a recurring theme throughout this book, and for good reason. Not only does it improve outcomes of treatment, reducing infections and complications, it's also so good for your mental health, managing stress, improving sleep - and it reduces your risk of recurrence. To paraphrase a remark said by many of the experts I spoke to over the course of my research: 'If the benefits of exercise were the result of a new drug that you could buy, it would be an enormous breakthrough in cancer treatment, and we'd hear about it all the time.'

Public health messaging has long tied exercise to weight loss, which can mean that people who don't need to lose weight feel that they don't need to exercise. And people who do want to lose weight often find a dispiriting lack of correlation between exercise and weight loss (because, as research has now shown, if you're eating processed foods and added sugar, you can't lose weight with exercise alone). Not only does this dated idea about exercise being the cure for obesity need to be thrown out, but also this public health strategy has been letting so many of us down for so long.

The latest research on the impact of physical activity on

breast cancer risk is from 2022 and was published in the *British Journal of Sports Medicine*. It involved data from more than 130,000 women, and clearly showed a causal effect between a sedentary lifestyle and breast cancer risk, strengthening the existing data on this, of which there is plenty.

'They've had trials of hundreds of thousands of patients who've been given prescription exercise, and it halves the risk of recurrence,' says Dr Liz O'Riordan. 'It also improves the physical and mental side effects of chemotherapy, radiotherapy and surgery. And it's just as important for the metastatic community because, by strengthening the bones and building up the muscles, it keeps you out of your bed for as long as possible. There's no evidence that it will slow the growth of the cancer, but it may have an effect on the immune system, making people more able to cope with the drugs they're having, so they can stay on them for longer.' She tells me that chemotherapy is often given even when the benefit is as low as 5 per cent. 'That means we believe it's worth giving 100 women chemotherapy to extend the lives of five. Exercise can extend the lives of 50, and it's free and there are no side effects. If you don't already, then, from the day you are diagnosed, you should start exercising because it will have an impact.'

So the evidence is extremely robust that, not only is movement one of the few things to be clinically proven to reduce your risk, but, even if you do have recurrence, being fit and strong will mean you have more treatment options and will be better placed to cope with it. I do wish that someone had told me about this sooner, because I basically lay on the sofa for a year after my diagnosis. With the weight of all this evidence, couldn't one of the doctors I met have mentioned moving my body a bit more? Why didn't they?

'Often, they don't know about it,' says Dr O'Riordan and, in response to my incredulous expression, she explains further. 'As a breast cancer surgeon, I would get four days a year to go to conferences. And those conferences were all about how to treat breast cancer, or the latest surgical techniques. I would assume that someone else was covering what I'd consider to be the softer stuff. You only know about it if you have a particular interest in that field. I didn't get any training on how to teach exercise to someone who's healthy, let alone someone with cancer. And it's one more thing to add to the consultation when you're only with your surgeon for half an hour.'

I get that time is an issue, but this is how I could have imagined that conversation going.

Doctor: 'Do you do much exercise?'

Me: 'No, I'm very lazy.'

Doctor: 'Well, it's been proven to improve the results of your treatment and reduce your risk of recurrence, so I'd highly recommend doing some. It makes a really big difference.'

I know there are people who need more support than a 30-second conversation to start incorporating more movement into their lives, and there is certainly lots of work to be done in that area. But, in the meantime, there are also lots of people who would do anything to reduce their risk of recurrence, and would have found it easy enough to make exercise a habit if only they knew just how important it is, particularly when compared with everything else.

Dr O'Riordan makes the point that, in an ideal world, there should be a contract between doctor and patient, in which doctors provide the best surgical and medical care, and the patient agrees to look after themselves with a healthy lifestyle including exercise, in order to get the best out of the treatment. She carried on exercising throughout her own cancer treatment in 2015, not because she was aware of any stats around exercise and cancer recurrence at that time but because she saw athletes on Twitter who were training through chemo. And she walked every day because other cancer patients had told her they felt it helped them. She was a fit, sporty person anyway, so was pleased to see that she could continue to do something that she enjoyed.

There are people like Dr Liz O'Riordan who will exercise naturally because they love it. Then there are people who are extremely resistant to exercise and will probably never do it, despite the consequences. They are at either end of the spectrum and, in the middle, there is a huge swathe of people like me, who don't have a natural inclination to exercise or weren't particularly sporty at school, and therefore haven't made it part of their adult life. I'd assume we're the majority, although I don't have stats on that. We're not necessarily averse to exercise; it's just always seemed a bit too much like hard work, and not necessarily for us. But we would absolutely do it if only we were given that information about how powerful it is for keeping you cancer-free. Anyway, I know now, and so do you, so no excuses.

What exactly should we be doing?

Sarah Newman is a cancer fitness specialist and founder of Get Me Back, an online community for women getting fit after cancer. She says that the recommendations for movement according to the World Health Organization are 150 minutes of moderate aerobic activity each week, which works out as around five 30-minute sessions. 'Think of something where you can just about hold a conversation, such as gardening, cleaning, brisk walking, chasing after the kids or going for a jog,' she says. 'Then you could try making around half of that time more vigorous cardio, where you're out of breath, such as running at a faster pace, cycling with hills or playing sport. After cancer treatment, this is a number to work up to, as it may not be possible right away.' So, if you're recovering from surgery or suffering with extreme fatigue during chemo, an amble around the block is fine. Anything is better than nothing.

On top of this aerobic activity, the recommendations suggest two strength or resistance sessions a week. 'That needs to be in there for bone and joint strength,' says Sarah. Make sure you have the sign-off from your surgical team before starting any strength training, and the important thing here is to build it up slowly. Sarah has an introduction to strength training on her YouTube channel @GetMeBackUK, as well as resistance band workouts for beginners. Getting a resistance band is a cheap and easy way to be able to do strength training at home.

If all this sounds too overwhelming or as if it's going to require too much organisation, then there are really simple ways that you can fit more movement into your life. Think of it as anything that works your muscles and amounts to an hour over the course of a week. Dr O'Riordan recommends a book called *Moving Through Cancer* by Dr Kathryn Schmitz, who shares lots of tips on getting your resistance training in when you don't feel as though you have the time or energy.

'It's things like, when the kettle's boiling, you do squats,' she explains. 'You do push-ups against the kitchen counter when the microwave's on. You do lunges when you're brushing your teeth. If you've got the washing to take upstairs, you do it one piece at a time. These are all simple body weight exercises that you can do at home throughout the day. You could have a resistance band and, when you're watching telly, do your shoulder exercises. You don't need to be in a gym.'

Some people love the structure, support and showy equipment of the gym environment, but it's definitely not for everyone. I've already mentioned that I now have a small dumbbell at home that I use whenever I get 10 minutes. I also learned that movement immediately after eating is a good way to balance blood sugar, so when I'm working from home I'll spend 10 minutes after lunch doing a few simple bicep curls or squats. It's quick, easy and free. For me, it works better than finding time to go to the gym for an hour.

If it's not raining, I try and do it in the garden, which gets a gold star from Sarah Newman. 'The benefits of being outside are genuinely proven to support your mental health as well as physical,' she says, 'so it's great to do your exercise outside.'

After breast cancer surgery, many women are anxious about weights, as often the only rehabilitation advice they're given is not to lift anything too heavy. But you can absolutely use weights. In fact, you should. Quite apart from the benefits in terms of reducing your risk of recurrence, weight training actually reduces your risk of lymphoedema and is great for strengthening your muscles and bones, which is particularly important after menopause.

Again, it's about starting slowly and building it up. If you like the gym, you can get support there, or you can learn through a breast cancer-specific online programme. Sarah Newman's online community Get Me Back also has an app. And there's a programme called Big Strong Lasses run by Carolyn Garritt, author of *Get Your Oomph Back*, a guide to exercise after cancer. Or have a chat with your GP who should be able to point you in the direction of local community initiatives. As long as you build it up slowly, you won't experience any adverse effects. But, if you feel like something isn't right, then stop immediately. As with so many steps in the process of rebuilding yourself, it's about listening to your body.

Joints

Listening to your body is also vital when it comes to your joints. This is true particularly of your knees, which require extra care after a post-cancer menopause. Many people love running, as much for the impact on their mind as on their body, but you might have a new anxiety about the impact on your knees. Reassuringly, research has shown that running causes the bone and cartilage to adapt, actually making knees stronger. The caveat to this is that overdoing it can cause harm, so don't go straight from being a non-runner to training for a marathon without giving your body time to adapt, and do get some good, supportive running shoes.

Get strong! Strength training the upper body

Sarah Newman's mission is to help you feel stronger and more in control, during and after cancer treatment. 'I have seen clients go from strength to strength, quite literally,' she says, 'by starting off using resistance bands and dumbbells, progressing to heavier kettlebells and even barbells, during and after treatment. I want to make strength training enjoyable so women feel empowered to keep it up. I'd always advise getting the go-ahead from your oncology team first and, ideally, receiving guidance from a cancer rehab specialist to advise on correct technique.'

She recommends following a few simple rules:

- Warm up and cool down before and after each workout.
- After surgery, nail shoulder mobility first, before lifting too much weight.
- When you're ready to begin lifting, start light and progress slowly.
- If you've had lymph node clearance, don't wrap resistance bands around the hands, avoid long (more than 45 seconds) static holds such as the plank, and allow for a rest day after strength training, but have a gentle walk to keep things moving.
- If you have lymphoedema, always wear your compression garment when exercising.
- Exercise to feel energised, not completely exhausted. This may mean a different level some days than others, and that's okay.

Strength exercises

Squat: Comparable to the movement of getting in and out of a chair. This simple but effective exercise can be

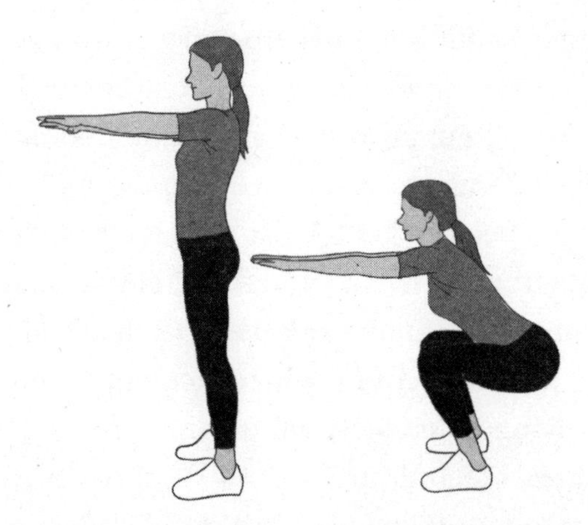

progressed by changing the level of support, resistance (i.e. by holding a weight or using a resistance band), range of motion or the way you position your legs. Start with a body weight 'sit to stand' from a chair, progress to taking the chair away, then using your body weight to squat, slowly adding weight to the movement.

Hinge: Effectively bending to pick something off the floor, but making sure you're using the right muscles and the correct form. Hinge movements like the deadlift can be tricky to master. I like to start using a pole. Stand in front of a mirror with your feet hip-width apart with a slight bend in the knee. Slide the pole down the front of the legs, pushing the bottom back, leaning your torso forward, maintaining a tight core and flat back. Then push into the floor and stand back up, pulling the pole with you and keeping the arms straight. This exercise can be progressed by holding weights.

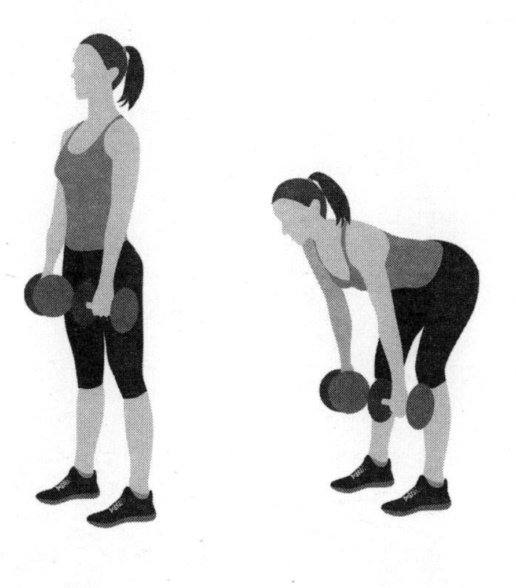

Push: Any exercise where you push weight or resistance away from you. An overhead press, or wall press-up, for example.

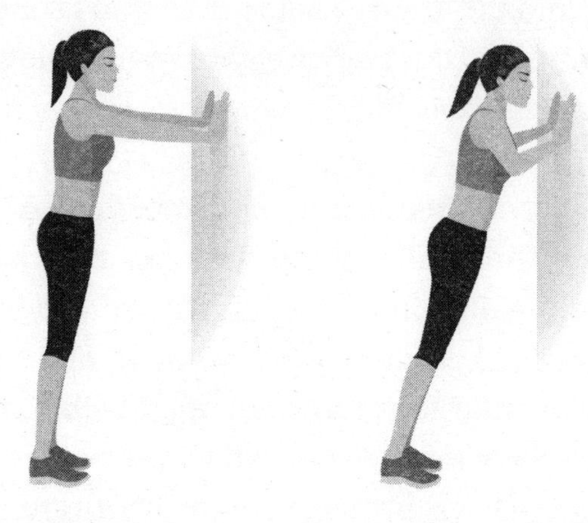

Pull: Movements where the effort of the exercise is the pull movement, such as an upright row, bent-over row or lat pull down. These are all great exercises to build strength and support good posture.

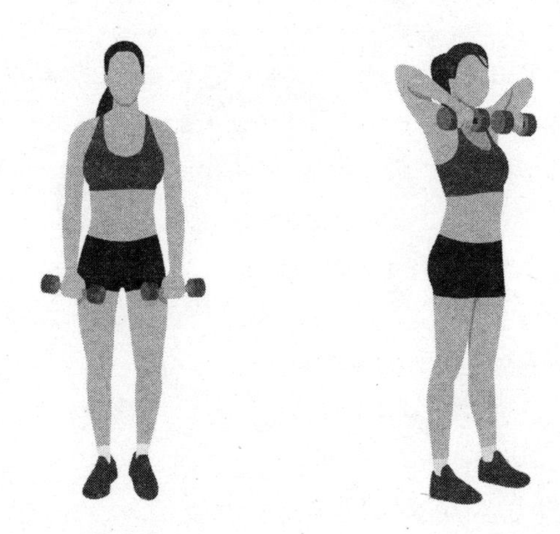

Lunge: A movement series that supports walking and stair climbing. Bad knees? Try a step up instead of a lunge.

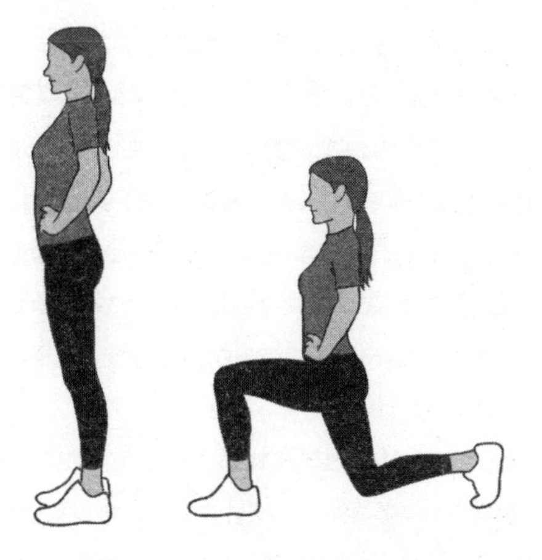

Find Sarah's videos on YouTube, and more specific advice at getmeback.uk.

Dance

If you can find a movement class that you enjoy, you'll have the added benefit of a sense of togetherness and community, which can increase optimism by helping you feel less isolated. Emily Jenkins is the founder of Move Dance Feel, a creative community that provides dance workshops for women affected by any type of cancer. She tells me that mental health benefits have been a powerful side effect of the classes, which most people initially attend for their physical health, with one participant describing it as 'a psychological game-changer'. The classes have been found to increase energy, improve mood, alleviate feelings of stress and anxiety, and liberate women from the gravity of having cancer.

'The outcomes in terms of improved confidence have been remarkable, resulting in women becoming more active in other ways,' says Emily. 'Joy manifests in dance, not only by feeling a sense of connection to others but also through feeling connected to ourselves, helping us to live in the present moment and free our minds from distracting or burdensome thoughts. With Move Dance Feel, this has led some women to feel calmer about their situation, and more reflective as to what is important in life.'

Another aspect of any kind of movement, but perhaps especially something as creative as dance, is getting back in touch with your own body. Cancer treatment can make you feel almost disassociated from your body – from the painful battery of tests to the mutilation of surgery and the way in which chemotherapy and hormonal treatments can leave us not looking or feeling like ourselves. Remember that what you've been through is a trauma, and a coping mechanism can be to separate your mind from what's happening in your body.

'Dancing helps women to regain trust in the body, and rediscover a new sense of body appreciation,' explains Emily. 'Making choices about how the body moves creatively also enables women to reclaim a sense of ownership of it. For many women this has been incredibly cathartic.' You will also get the best kind of positive feedback, as you feel your body getting stronger, with increased balance and stability.

Yoga

In a similar way to dance, you'll often hear of people getting into yoga after cancer treatment, which makes sense to me because the benefits of yoga are as much for your mind as your body. Marcia Mercier is a yoga teacher with a specialist focus on yoga for breast cancer, having been through her own diagnosis when she was 32.

'It's such a trauma to your body,' she says now. 'It turns your whole world upside down.' Her children were two and four at the time, so, like many of us, she held it together for their benefit during treatment. But it was when treatment ended that she really struggled. 'That's when it really hit me,' she says. 'You get through it and then, when it's all over, you think you should be elated. You expect to be celebrating but, actually, you don't feel like that at all. I felt overwhelmed by what I'd been through. I was trying to get back to normal, but I found that I wasn't my usual self. I was irritable, easily stressed and on the verge of tears most of the time.'

Eventually she went to the doctor, who suggested she go for counselling, but she didn't feel she wanted to do that. On a whim, she decided to try a yoga class, not knowing much about it other than hearing about the benefits for body and mind. 'It wasn't a special yoga for cancer class or anything, it was just at the local gym, but it actually made me feel good in my body,' she says. 'It made me feel I was regaining strength. It felt calming and centring, and addressed the body holistically, not just the physical. I didn't know how it was working. But it was working.'

Marcia went on to learn about the science of yoga, and the ways in which it can help address a lot of the side effects of breast cancer treatment. She describes how yogic breathing techniques can regulate the nervous system, and how moving between yoga poses along with the breath can have a profound effect on your circulation and lymphatic flow. Her classes – which she runs online as well as in person at Future Dreams House in London – are for anyone going through or recovering from cancer treatment.

Adaptable around your PICC line or port during treatment, and modified for any physical limitations after surgery, her classes are designed to energise the body and soothe the nervous system. This is why specific yoga for cancer classes are brilliant; it's so good for you during cancer treatment, but it's also a time when going to a normal yoga class can feel scary and intimidating. Marcia's classes at Future Dreams House are one of several breast cancer-specific exercise classes held there, including ones with yoga-for-cancer specialist Vicky Fox which are also available to stream online if you're based elsewhere in the country.

'There is more and more research out there now, indicating that exercise pre-treatment, during and post-treatment is really beneficial in terms of managing side effects and helping you recover more quickly,' says Marcia. 'So try to carry on with a gentle yoga practice or another exercise throughout treatment, if you can. Of course there are going to be weeks when you're not going to feel up to even getting on a mat, and that's absolutely fine. It's about listening to your body. Yoga is much more than the poses; a simple breathing practice is still yoga.'

Bringing awareness is such a key element of yoga, and it's one that affects every area of your life, not just your body. 'The way in which yoga comes into your life is not only on the mat,' she explains. 'You actually become more aware of the choices that you make. It eventually has a positive impact on what you eat, what you drink, how you carry yourself throughout your day. It has a much wider reach than just that hour that you spend in the yoga class.'

Pilates

Many yoga studios offer mat Pilates classes. However, if you can find one with reformer machines, then reformer Pilates is one of the best forms of rehab that you can do post-surgery. Combining strength training with stretches, it can improve everything from flexibility and posture, to balance - which is so important after menopause as your bones are not as strong and improving balance will reduce your risk of falls.

One thing that I particularly love about it is that you really have to focus during the class, paying attention to each movement and how the machine works with you. This leaves little headspace for spiralling anxiety or dark post-cancer fears. It also actually feels really good in your body, as the resistance of the machine stretches you right out. Take it from someone who has never really considered themselves an exercise person - reformer Pilates is a hard yes from me.

As with many elements of future-proofing your body, there is crossover between the sections of this book. Yoga and Pilates are here under 'Movement', but could just as easily appear in the chapter about stress. The power of a practice that incorporates breathing with movement to soothe your nervous system is extremely good for your mind. It can be one of the most useful tools in your toolbox and, let's face it, during cancer treatment you will very likely need the whole box.

Sticking with it

Starting a new exercise programme is one thing, sticking with it is quite another. Remind yourself that it's much easier to maintain a streak than it is to start a habit back up again once you've let it lapse. Accountability strategies can really help with fighting the inclination to jack it all in when you don't feel up to it. Try roping in a friend to join you for a regular walk, or joining an online fitness community such as Get Me Back.

If you really feel like you don't know where to start in terms of becoming more active, CanRehab is an amazing organisation that matches cancer patients to an instructor who can provide a number of sessions tailored to the person's needs, based on their stage of treatment and previous exercise experience. They're developing a register of approved personal trainers and health professionals qualified to provide programmes for people living with or recovering from cancer, and have now trained more than 700 fitness and health professionals throughout the UK. CanRehab started out by supporting SafeFit, a research trial showing the enormous benefits of movement for anyone with cancer.

Interestingly, all of this research is really quite new. It was only in 2007 that CanRehab founder Professor Anna Campbell published the results of a study showing that it was safe and effective for women diagnosed with breast cancer to exercise during chemotherapy and radiotherapy. This study was one of the first to demonstrate how to deliver a community exercise programme for people with cancer, as it was based on circuit classes taking place in local council leisure centres.

Things are slowly starting to change, and movement will hopefully soon be taken seriously as part of cancer care, but there are still obstacles to overcome. On one hand, some patients just don't want to hear it, which I understand. 'It's hard work,' says Dr Liz O'Riordan. 'As a doctor you're basically saying: "I'm going to make you postmenopausal, which will make you put on weight, and you're going to hate yourself, and then I'm going to tell you that you've got to lose the weight, you've got to stop drinking and you've got to exercise . . ." That's no fun. It's really hard getting the message across positively.'

Then there's the less understandable resistance from medical professionals. Dr O'Riordan describes her struggle to get her own hospital to promote 5k Your Way, an initiative to encourage people with cancer to walk, run, cheer or volunteer at a local Parkrun event once a month. 'It's ridiculous,' she says with a sigh. 'There's still this barrier. I don't know what it is. But if we can get patients asking, "Why aren't you telling me about exercise? What can I do?" then doctors might realise that they've been missing a trick.'

As with all areas of health, everybody is different. You only have to look at a class of children to see that some people are naturally sporty and truly find their joy through running, swimming, team sports or athletics. Meanwhile, others have less of a natural inclination towards movement. As I've mentioned, I'm in this category – yes, I was the girl that hid in the toilets on sports day because I hated it so much. If you're the same, it doesn't mean that we're lazy. But it does mean that we have to make more of an effort to incorporate movement into our lives, because it might not come naturally. There *will* be something out there that you find you actually enjoy doing, whether that's cycling, walking, dancing – even housework and DIY count.

It's easy to get caught up in whether or not you're doing the right kind of exercise, but the truth is, the best kind of exercise is the one that you will actually practise regularly. Don't force yourself to do a type of exercise that you hate, because that's counterproductive when you're trying to learn how to feel better about yourself after cancer treatment. You might be surprised about where it leads and how good it makes you feel to use your body well, potentially for the first time in your adult life. You might even become fitter and stronger than you were pre-diagnosis. This can be a moment for seriously positive change.

Nutrition

It is often claimed that Hippocrates said: 'Let food be thy medicine and medicine be thy food.' Whether he did or didn't, considering he was around in about 400 BC he didn't have much choice in the matter. Almost two-and-a-half thousand years later, we can pop a painkiller for a headache, take antibiotics for an infection and have chemo for our cancer.

This is all brilliant, of course, but I'd argue that we shouldn't allow it to let us lose sight of the power of food to transform how we feel. The trouble is, this power has been co-opted by certain sections of the wellness world to sell products or push a certain ideology.

If you're a person with an interest in nutrition, or even if you're not, then you probably already know how overwhelming this world can be. There are mountains of conflicting advice and information out there, and so many very vocal proponents of a particular dietary doctrine or other, making it hard to separate fact from fiction.

Let's look at what we *do* know for sure. The World Cancer Research Fund (WCRF) and the American Institute for Cancer Research have created a series of guidelines produced by panels of expert scientists reviewing the evidence from thousands of scientific papers. The report has been endorsed by the World Health Organization and, although the majority of the research is about preventing cancer in the first place rather than reducing your risk of recurrence, it's still the most reliable information out there. They produced the following recommendations, with the caveat that people should treat them as a package of lifestyle choices, rather than picking or choosing from the list:

1. Keep your weight within the healthy range, and avoid weight gain.
2. Be physically active every day; walk more and sit less.
3. Eat whole grains, vegetables, fruit and beans as part of your usual diet.
4. Limit fast foods and other processed foods high in saturated fat or sugar.
5. Limit red meat and eat little, if any, processed meat.
6. Drink water and limit sugar-sweetened drinks.
7. Limit alcohol consumption.
8. Aim to meet your nutritional needs through diet alone, rather than using supplements.

I'm not going to argue with any of these points, partly because that would be arguing with really quite robust research. And partly because it's largely common sense: we all know that we should have more fruit, veg and water, and less sugar, booze and processed foods.

But I am going to say that I don't feel comfortable with the first point stipulating a 'healthy range' of weight, because that is so vague and, if it's referring to the BMI (body mass index) system that categorises a large number of British people as obese, then it's not that helpful. If you tell someone that smoking, drinking or eating processed foods increases your risk of cancer, then it's pretty clear what you need to do in those situations in order to reduce your risk. Citing obesity or 'weight gain' as a risk factor, however, is much less clear. The public health obsession with 'tackling obesity' does nothing but make people feel bad about themselves, largely because obesity is tied to identity. You say a person 'is obese' but you would never say a person 'is' cancer. They 'have' cancer. Anyway, there are many factors that contribute to the size and shape of a person's body, including genetics, hormonal balance, blood sugar levels and environment, so simply telling someone that they ought to lose weight is too simplistic an approach.

Also, if your only goal is weight loss, then it can paradoxically lead to unhealthy behaviours. I've known people obsessed with calories that won't eat avocados or nuts because they're too calorie-dense and, if they're going out, they don't eat all day to save their calories for booze. That is mad to me, and is clearly not helping reduce your risk of cancer.

Rather than focusing on obesity as the enemy, could we focus on the things that might lead to such high rates of obesity in the UK? School dinners and hospital meals would be a good place to start. As someone with experience of both over the last few years, I can attest that they are doing nothing to improve the health of the nation. My kids come back from school every day talking about the ice cream, cake or jelly they had for dessert at lunchtime. And, when I was in hospital for my mastectomy, I was quite shocked at what was on the menu. One morning, I asked if they had any plain yoghurt for breakfast. No, they only had flavoured yoghurt. If I wanted a healthy option, I could have the fat-free one, they suggested, gesturing to a fluorescent-coloured, sugar-packed processed yoghurt.

Anyway, despite my discomfort with talking about obesity,

I do understand that facts are facts, and it is a fact that obesity has now overtaken smoking to become the leading cause of cancer in the UK. Dr Liz O'Riordan believes there is a way to address it without banging on about 'tackling obesity'.

'It's about maintaining a healthy weight, whatever that is for you,' she says, with emphasis on the second part of that sentence. 'I generally say around a size 14 to 16, to give people an idea. Because it's not just about being overweight: it's how the whole immune system and the chemicals in your body work when you are obese. The answer is eating a healthy well-balanced diet, with mainly a rainbow of fruit and veg, to keep your immune system strong and healthy. It's hard work and it's boring,' she adds, which is not quite the attitude with which I asked you to go into this process, but it is reassuring to learn that even a super-fit breast cancer doctor sometimes finds healthy living hard and boring.

A more positive way to look at nutrition is to consider the enormous benefits it can have on your mood and mental health. You might have heard of the SMILES trial (Supporting the Modification of lifestyle in Lowered Emotional States), the results of which were published in 2017. They showed that a Mediterranean-style diet based on whole grains, plant foods and good quality meat, fish and dairy reduced depressive symptoms over a three-month period, to the extent that a third of those in the dietary support group met criteria for remission of major depression. It's a truly groundbreaking result, proving that what we eat impacts not only our physical health but also our emotional wellbeing.

Eat the rainbow

You will have heard people talk about 'eating the rainbow', which simply means ensuring you eat a variety of different-coloured plant foods. There are many reasons for that. Not only do they contain large amounts of fibre, vitamins and minerals, they're also full of phytonutrients: natural compounds that protect plants from bugs, germs and fungi. Eating phytonutrients affects your cellular structure and can help prevent disease and keep your body functioning at its best. And it's easier than you might think to improve the variety of different-coloured plants that you eat. You don't have to source a purple carrot from a specialist retailer. Here's a handy list to consider next time you do the weekly shop:

RED: tomatoes, red pepper, watermelon, pomegranate, apples, chilli, lentils.

ORANGE: carrot, apricot, mango, pumpkin, squash, sweet potato, peaches, clementines.

GREEN: kale, spinach, courgette, green beans, broccoli, celery, avocados, apples, peas.

PURPLE: blueberries, aubergine, beetroot, red grapes, plums, kidney beans, dates.

WHITE: cauliflower, leeks, potatoes, oats, garlic, butter beans, chickpeas.

Do certain foods prevent or cause cancer?

You might read articles claiming that certain foods have been shown to cause cancer, but that information is almost always a wilful misinterpretation of the research. 'There is no one food that causes breast cancer recurrence,' explains Dr O'Riordan. 'Dairy is fine, soya is fine. You don't need to be vegan. Processed meat has been shown to increase your risk of breast cancer, but that would be if you were eating sausages and bacon every day. Everything in moderation is fine.'

As for foods that can reduce your risk of cancer, there really is no silver bullet, despite what you might read about superfoods. 'If you eat healthily in general, you don't need to worry about superfoods,' says Dr O'Riordan. 'If people are eating a really bad diet in general, then a superfood smoothie of wheatgrass and ginseng and blueberries is going to make them feel great because they're getting all these vitamins and minerals, which they're not normally.'

So, ideally, you would be getting everything you need from a healthy and varied diet with plenty of different-coloured vegetables. But we've all had weeks when we're on a deadline, or on holiday, or it's the run-up to Christmas and we've not been eating as well as we should. In those instances, I do think a superfood smoothie certainly has its place even if normally you shouldn't need it.

Mushrooms

One food that is often talked about as a wonder cure when it comes to cancer prevention is mushrooms. You don't have to spend long on social media (in cancer circles, anyway) to see someone claiming that mushrooms shrank their cancer – usually with a discount code so you can buy an expensive supplement.

'It's bullshit,' says Dr O'Riordan, frankly. 'People believe influencers who have hundreds of thousands of followers and that's the problem. You assume that someone is telling you the truth, and then you feel like, "Oh my god, I got breast cancer because I didn't eat mushrooms." But there is no special diet that has been shown to cure or prevent cancer.'

People will cite research about the efficacy of mushrooms but, as Dr O'Riordan explains, it's all been laboratory-based (i.e. with cancer cells in a petri dish, which is very different to the human body) or animal-based at best.

'What they have not done,' she says, 'is get a load of cancer patients and say: "Right, you're going to have chemo and you're going to have mushrooms and let's see who dies first." You could say that trial is never going to happen. But, even if you did monitor people who eat more mushrooms (in an observational trial), the chances are that those people have a healthier diet overall. They're eating mushrooms, so they're probably eating other vegetables and looking after themselves. How can you say it's the mushrooms? It's a bit like saying, people who smoke get lung cancer, and people who smoke drink coffee, so therefore coffee causes lung cancer. That's the trouble with observational studies, because there are so many other factors. You can have a 20-page study and just pick one sentence out to highlight whatever you want to take out of context.'

The official line on mushrooms from Cancer Research UK is this: 'There is currently not enough evidence that any type of mushroom can prevent or cure cancer.'[5] Although some compounds found in mushrooms have been shown to stop or slow the growth of cancer cells in laboratory studies, they state, 'we have to be cautious about such early research. Substances that can kill cells in laboratory conditions don't necessarily turn out to be useful treatments in people.' Yes, there have been trials where mushrooms are prescribed alongside cancer treatment, and seem to reduce side effects and improve overall outcomes. But proving a reduction in cancer risk would involve a large trial over many years, costing millions, so that has not happened.

Having said that, mushrooms are used in Japan and China to treat lung diseases, where they are often given alongside cancer treatment. Research here in the UK is looking at whether mushrooms can help the immune system and, if they do, if this could help fight cancer cells.

Also, acknowledging there is no magic single ingredient shouldn't mean dismissing nutrient-rich foods altogether. It's pretty clear that mushrooms have many benefits – such as vitamins, polyphenols, fibre and prebiotics. They have also been shown to absorb vitamin D from the sun through their skin and so are an excellent natural source of the vitamin, which many scientists believe is far more bioavailable (in other words, able to be used by the body) than synthetic supplements. So you should eat them if you like them. I personally don't like them but, in an effort to eat a wider variety of vegetables in general, I am forcing myself to keep trying, and can now just about tolerate them if they're chopped up very small.

Anti-angiogenesis

Although it's true that there is no single food or nutrient that can compensate for a generally poor diet, I do believe that there are some particularly powerful and nutrient-dense foods that it's worth making an effort to include, regardless of how well you eat otherwise.

Dr William Li is the author of *Eat to Beat Disease: The New Science of How Your Body Can Heal Itself*. He agrees that a healthy diet overall is vital, particularly for anyone who has been through cancer treatment. 'First, there is the repair of damaged tissues from the treatment itself that must be achieved,' he explains. 'While the body will restore itself, what you eat can help speed this along. Second is the need to shore up your internal defences to lower the risk of the cancer coming back.'

He says it's possible to do this by preventing blood vessels from feeding cancer cells. This is called 'anti-angiogenesis'. Cancer cells don't start out with a blood supply, he explains. This is why they appear and disappear harmlessly in healthy people, because they are not receiving oxygen or nutrients. This explains why autopsies of people who died in car accidents showed that about 40 per cent of women between the ages of 40 and 50 have microscopic cancers in their breasts. The problem arises when those cancer cells get their own blood supply and become a growing tumour.

So what does he recommend to encourage this process of anti-angiogenesis? 'Green tea, soya, tomatoes and leafy greens have been shown to help do this,' he says. 'There are also foods that kill cancer stem cells, the deadly cells responsible for a cancer's return. Remarkably, matcha tea has been shown in lab studies to kill breast cancer stem cells.' Here, I can't help thinking of Dr Liz O'Riordan's warning that laboratory studies are not the same as human studies but, still, I like matcha green tea so I'll keep drinking it, with measured optimism about its health benefits.

Dr Li also recommends kiwi, watermelon and citrus for protecting against certain DNA mutations, and mushrooms, nuts, blueberries and pomegranate for supporting your immune defences. In his 2010 TED Talk, *Can We Eat To Starve Cancer?* he lists many other foods that have this effect, including what you might already think of as 'anticancer' foods such as green tea and turmeric, but also many day-to-day foods including apples, oranges, lemons, kale, tomato, garlic, parsley and olive oil.

I ask him if there should be a different approach for triple negative versus hormone receptor positive cancers, when it comes to diet, but he says not. 'The power is in activating your body's health defences that combat cancer,' he explains. 'Starving a tumour and lowering inflammation is beneficial for any type of breast cancer. Lowering DNA mutation rates and unleashing tumour suppressor genes is protective against multiple forms of cancer. And a heightened immunity is also part of your body's natural shield.'

Now, I know that lots of people bristle at the term 'starve cancer', considering it vague and unscientific, but I do believe in Dr Li's work around how food can support your immune system to work as best as it can. Particularly since what he recommends is in keeping with general advice about healthy eating anyway: eat a wide variety of different-coloured plants and avoid highly processed foods.

Sugar

We can't talk about starving cancer without discussing sugar. When I was first diagnosed, several people told me that I should cut sugar out of my diet entirely, since 'cancer cells feed on sugar' and, to an extent, that's true. But – predictably, as with everything to do with nutrition – it's not as straightforward as that. Yes, cancer cells do consume glucose, but it would be neither realistic nor advisable to avoid all glucose. It's naturally occurring in many fruits, vegetables and whole grains, all of which are good for you.

The issue, as I learned during my experience with PCOS in my 20s, occurs when your blood sugar spikes dramatically. This tends not to happen with naturally occurring sugars in fruit and veg because it is tempered by the plant fibre. So added refined sugars are the thing to avoid, for many reasons (from your mood to your hormones to your teeth). But, if you crave sweet things, there are ways that you can manage blood sugar spikes to improve your energy and support your immunity. These include eating your vegetables and protein first, rather than having sugar on an empty stomach, and doing some kind of movement such as going for a walk after eating.

Glucose monitors – once the preserve of diabetics only – have become popular with people who enjoy monitoring their health statistics, along with sleep trackers and heart rate variability technology. You no longer have to prick your finger because you can now buy continuous glucose monitors that come as a small water-resistant sensor with a tiny probe that is placed on the back of the arm and monitors your blood sugar levels every 60 seconds. If you want to give it a go, you'll learn a lot about how your body responds to certain foods.

But you can mostly use your common sense to avoid blood sugar spikes.

Gut health

Another reason to avoid added sugars and refined carbohydrates (which act like sugar in your blood stream) is that your gut bacteria are not fans. Having beneficial bacteria in the gut helps with many functions of the body and mind, including digestion, balancing your mood, reducing anxiety, protecting against infections and – some people claim – cancer. Keeping your microbiome thriving is all about balance, and ensuring healthy growth of good gut bacteria while minimising bad bacteria. This is why antibiotics should generally be avoided unless absolutely necessary, because they kill bacteria indiscriminately, including the good guys. Your good bacteria can also be inhibited by stress, surgery, illness, trauma or unhealthy eating habits. If you've had a cancer diagnosis, the first four of those are pretty unavoidable unfortunately, so you might as well give all you've got to the latter element – what you eat.

'Feeding your healthy gut bacteria reduces inflammation, which is a trigger for cancer growth and regrowth,' says Dr Li. 'So prebiotics and probiotics can be helpful.'

Probiotics are the bacteria themselves, and they're found in live yoghurt, kefir, sauerkraut, miso, kimchi and kombucha. Prebiotics are what the bacteria feed on, and they include garlic, onions, leeks, asparagus, Jerusalem artichoke, oats, apples and basically anything with lots of fibre, so most fruit and veg. In fact, the things that are good for your gut are very similar to the things that are good for all other aspects of health: eat a wide variety of fibre-rich plant foods, including pulses and legumes, nuts, seeds, herbs, whole grains, fruits, and tonnes of vegetables (there is really no such thing as too much veg when it comes to eating healthily). Limit or avoid processed foods and those high in added sugar, and drink plenty of water.

Fasting

In recent years, a lot of attention has been focused on fasting as a way to improve your gut health and your general well-being. It's also something that comes up a lot when talking about cancer and nutrition. While there is no hard evidence to prove that it's effective in reducing your risk of recurrence, it certainly seems like a good thing to do for general health. We now know that your digestive system needs time to recover between meals in order to function as it should. Intermittent fasting, or time-restricted eating, means eating dinner early and breakfast later, with a 12–16 hour 'fast' in between (much of which you're asleep for, which makes it easier). This is something that I do, and I certainly feel healthier for it, but it could be mostly because being strict about when I stop eating in the evening has put an end to late-night snacking.

There is some evidence that fasting around chemotherapy infusions potentially improves the response to treatment by repairing DNA damage in normal tissue and increasing tumour cells' sensitivity to chemo. More human studies with adequate sample sizes and follow-ups are required to confirm these findings, but this is one of those approaches that doesn't appear to have a downside, so it's worth trying.

'Fasting helps to "re-boot" the systems your body uses to counter cancer,' explains Dr Li. 'It is beneficial for the gut microbiome, which leads to an anti-inflammatory response, and it can help to optimise your immune system. Fasting also reverses the effect of the common practice of overloading the body with calories. Overeating strains your metabolism as well as health defences, making you more vulnerable to a host of diseases, including cancer.'

So, while there is a certain amount of evidence around fasting, I don't think you need to take it to extremes. Perhaps the simple aim of cutting out snacking after dinner in the evening could be doable? That would give your digestive system a break, and not eating too late also improves your sleep. Then don't worry too much about what time you have breakfast. Your focus should really be on the quality of food that you're eating, rather than sticking to a particular rigid schedule.

Eat seasonally

One of the best things that you can do for your nutritional health is to eat with the seasons. Human beings have evolved over hundreds of thousands of years to eat seasonally. Before we had fruit flown over from the other side of the world, we ate whatever grew at that time of year. Now I'm not saying never eat a banana because they don't grow in the UK. I'm happy to take advantage of modern advances that allow us to eat a variety of fresh fruits and vegetables all year round. But the less the food has to travel to reach you, the fresher it will be, and therefore more nutritious and delicious. It's also significantly better for the environment, and just a nicer way to eat because you have the reassuring predictability of asparagus season arriving in spring, or warming root-vegetable stews as the months get colder.

In an ideal world, we'd all be like my mum, who grows her own veg, feasting on broad beans, tomatoes, peas and spring greens all summer. She even keeps bags of potatoes that she dug up in the autumn in her shed, which then last all winter. But realistically, most of us are not going to do that. A good alternative is to book a regular delivery of an organic veg box. There are big companies that do this nationwide, such as Abel & Cole, Riverford or Odd Box, but it's also worth checking for small local initiatives, which are often cheaper and even more sustainable.

The great thing about doing this is that it forces you to get creative when you have no idea what to do with, for example, a large bunch of beetroot. (It turns out beetroot grows pretty much all year round in the UK, so we've certainly learned a few variations on beetroot burgers, beetroot risotto and beetroot soup in our house.) The downside is that on those weeks when you're too busy to work out what to do with it, you might have a bunch of beetroot decaying in the bottom of your fridge.

A good way to start is to look at what's in season now and choose something that you like from that list. There are lots of lists online, notably on the Vegetarian Society website (vegsoc.org) and at the self-explanatory eattheseasons.co.uk. There are also some lovely cookery books designed around seasonal eating, such as Gill Meller's *Time: A Year and a Day in the Kitchen* and *The Modern Cook's Year* by Anna Jones.

This is not an exhaustive list, but here's a cut-out-and-keep guide to when the most common British-grown fruit and veg is in season.

January/February

Apples, Carrots, Celery, Kale, Leeks, Mushrooms, Parsnips, Pears, Red Cabbage, Squash, Swedes, Turnips, White Cabbage.

March/April

Artichoke, Beetroot, Carrots, Leeks, Purple Sprouting Broccoli, Radishes, Rhubarb, Spring Onions, New Potatoes, Kale, Rocket, Spinach.

May/June

Asparagus, Peppers, Broad Beans, Lettuce, New Potatoes, Radishes, Rhubarb, Rocket, Spinach, Strawberries, Broccoli, Cherries, Courgettes, Cucumber, Peas, Runner Beans.

July/August

Blackberries, Fennel, French Beans, Summer Squash, Sweetcorn, Aubergine, Cherries, Courgettes, Cucumber, Peas, Samphire, Strawberries, Mangetout, Tomatoes.

September/October

Damsons, Garlic, Plums, Wild Mushrooms, Butternut Squash, Cauliflower, Onions, Potatoes, Pumpkin, Red Cabbage, Samphire, Tomatoes, Watercress.

November/December

Brussels Sprouts, Celeriac, Winter Squash, Chestnuts, Cranberries, Jerusalem Artichokes, Leeks, Parsnips, Savoy Cabbage, Swiss Chard.

Nutrients to include in your diet

It's easy to become stressed and obsessed with nutrition, and I don't want you to get caught up in whether or not you're getting enough of one specific nutrient or another. Having said that, it can be helpful to have a handy list of things to try and include in your diet, if you like them. As well as the above lists of different-coloured fruit and veg and seasonal foods, this is a list I have stuck inside my kitchen cupboard door at home. If there's a food on here that I haven't tried in a while, I'll add it to the shopping order and try to include it at some point soon. It's not about exclusion or denial; it's about inclusion and enjoyment.

So much of eating well is about your attitude towards food. You should enjoy what you eat, embrace the challenge of eating a wider variety of whole foods and have fun experimenting with new things and different ways to cook them. Even if you hate cooking, or have ingrained ideas about healthy food being boring, try and make a conscious choice to think of it in a more positive way. I always used to say that I hated exercise, but I've forced myself to try out different things and now I actually enjoy it. Overcoming years of conditioning about your attitude towards food won't change overnight but, as with anything, you more you do it the easier it becomes. Hopefully this list will help you with that. Don't think of it as a rigid guide of what to eat – there's so much on here, that would simply be overwhelming. It's more to inspire you to try and include a wide range of healthy foods.

- **Vitamin K** has been shown to have cancer-fighting properties (in a petri dish at least), and vitamin K-rich foods are good for you in many other ways too, so it's worth stocking up on spinach, kale, broccoli, cabbage, asparagus, avocado and lime.
- **Flavonoids** are often hailed as an 'anticancer' compound, and they're found in red and purple fruits and vegetables, including cherries, raspberries, beetroot, grapes, pomegranates and plums.
- **Vitamin D** is vital for immunity and difficult to absorb from food, so sunlight is the most important source, but you can also find it in eggs, mushrooms and oily fish.
- **Whole grains** are far better for you than processed, refined versions. Try oats, brown rice, quinoa and buckwheat.
- **Legumes** have a host of health benefits, particularly as a source of protein, so try and include chickpeas, butter beans, black beans, kidney beans and lentils.
- **Omega-3 fatty acids** are great for your brain and joints, and researchers are currently studying the effects of them on delaying or reducing tumour development in breast and prostate cancer. Find them in oily fish like mackerel, salmon and tuna. Plant-based sources include flaxseeds, walnuts and chia seeds.
- **Anti-inflammatory foods** will help prevent low-level chronic inflammation, which is caused by inactivity, ultra-processed foods and refined sugars and can result in heart disease, type 2 diabetes, certain cancers, digestive issues, arthritis and various brain disorders. Good anti-inflammatory foods include turmeric, garlic, berries, almonds, broccoli and those all-powerful dark green leafy vegetables.

- **Antioxidants**. Get your vitamins A, C and E from sweet potato, carrots, red pepper, oranges, strawberries, broccoli, nuts and seeds.
- **Protein** is obviously in meat, fish and eggs, but plant-based sources are important if you don't eat much meat. Try quinoa, beans, lentils, nuts and seeds.
- **Herbs and spices** are delicious and so good for you. Experiment with ginger, cinnamon, chilli, paprika, peppermint, oregano, rosemary, cumin, coriander and so many others.
- **Turmeric** deserves its own entry, even though it's a spice with which most of us are already familiar. It contains an active chemical called curcumin, which has been shown to destroy cancer cells in some promising early trials. More research is needed but, in the meantime, Cancer Research UK advises against mega-dosing with curcumin capsules. However, cooking with reasonable amounts of turmeric, may do you a world of good, and makes curries taste great.

Organic vs non-organic

This is another area where people have strong views, either claiming we should buy all-organic or claiming that organic food is a pointless rip-off. Perhaps predictably, I'm somewhere in the middle. As I understand it, there is no hard clinical evidence proving a correlation between pesticides on our food and risk of developing cancer. But it makes sense to me that reducing our exposure to toxic chemicals can only help, right?

I tend to buy organic eggs and dairy products because I (perhaps misguidedly) believe it's better for the animals. And

I buy organic fruit and veg when my family and I would be eating the skin that has been exposed to pesticides, such as apples, berries, grapes, peppers, celery, kale, potatoes and tomatoes. But I don't bother buying organic if it's something where we remove the skin before eating it, such as bananas, pineapple, melon and avocados.

It's easy to become overwhelmed by all the information out there, or feel pressured by anyone who claims you need to eat a certain way. But it's really very simple. As the World Cancer Research Fund's recommendations state, eat a variety of plants, while reducing refined sugars and ultra-processed foods. I'd probably add to their list that you should focus on fibre for gut health, think about balancing your blood sugar, learn to love cooking from scratch with fresh ingredients, experiment with herbs and spices, eat the rainbow and, most importantly of all, enjoy it!

Supplements

Generally, like the WCRF, I don't approve of supplements because I believe it's better to get nutrients from food. My exceptions to this rule are:

- To correct a deficiency such as iron, when your doctor has said that you need to.
- An omega-3 supplement if you don't eat fish, since plant-based sources are not as complete, meaning you'd have to eat a *lot* of walnuts and flaxseeds to get enough.
- B vitamin complex if you're vegan, since B12 in particular is found in meat, fish, eggs and dairy products.

- A probiotic if you're recovering from an infection or have had antibiotics.
- Everyone in the northern hemisphere should be taking a vitamin D supplement in the winter, particularly if you have darker skin.

One of the main issues I have with supplements is that the industry is not regulated, so you could spend a lot of money on fillers and bulking agents. Also, having too much of a particular vitamin or nutrient can be as bad for you as having too little of it.

Over the course of my career as a journalist, I have spoken to many experts and nutritionists about supplements, but it's hard to find one who isn't on the payroll of a supplements brand, so have somewhat of a vested interest.

Dr Liz O'Riordan is extremely cynical about claims made by the supplement industry, saying that, other than in some instances where supplementation is recommended by a doctor, often what people actually need is a good night's sleep and some vegetables.

'People want an easy fix,' she says. 'The basic truth is it's about eating a healthy diet, not drinking a lot of alcohol, exercising and drinking water. It's not exciting, it's not sexy. But, if something seems too good to be true, it probably is. And if someone is making money from it, or if a celebrity's got a discount code on social media, I would say: can you find three other people who aren't being paid by that company, who also agree that this works? Is it really worth spending time and money on this? If it makes you feel great, then that's fine, but you probably don't need it.'

Having said all of that, I am quite interested in mushroom supplements. I know, I know, Dr O'Riordan would roll her eyes. But as I said earlier there do appear to be a range of health benefits to be gained from mushrooms and, since I don't like them, I'm not getting those benefits.

'Medicinal mushrooms' like reishi and lion's mane are used pretty widely in Asian countries and, in Japan for example, mushroom polysaccharides have been approved for use in the public healthcare system since 1984 as part of integrative therapy for digestive cancers. There are also clinical trials into the efficacy of medicinal mushrooms happening in Spain. Toral Shah is a nutritional scientist, functional medicine practitioner and founder of theurbankitchen.co.uk. She has a BSc in cell biology and an MSc in nutritional medicine. Having been through breast cancer herself, Toral has a special interest in reducing the risk of recurrence. I asked her what she takes and her answer was . . . a mushroom supplement.

So, while they're not cheap, I have to admit that I buy them on a sporadic basis. Other than that, I tend to dip in and out of supplements covering common deficiencies.

Magnesium is known as 'nature's valium', but rather than pop a pill, you can absorb it through your skin in the form of an Epsom salt bath. The bath will arguably relax your nervous system as much as the magnesium, so it's win-win.

Then I'll occasionally try a supergreens powder in my smoothie, or I'll take some of those digestive health shots for a few weeks. So, yes, I dabble. But it's important to mention that I'm in the extremely fortunate position of working in an industry where I am sometimes sent supplements to try out. Some of them I like so much that I have since bought top-ups. These include The Turmeric Co. immunity shots, Symprove for gut health, and Hifas da Terra for mushroom extracts. Others have gone straight in the bin: please don't send me your sugar-packed gummies, I see right through them.

But before you dabble, I highly recommend you first focus on good nutrition, managing stress, staying physically active, getting enough sleep and connecting with others in a meaningful way. Think about the 'low-hanging fruit' of wellness; the things that you can fairly easily incorporate into your life on a daily basis. Get your health fundamentals right and you won't need to spend money on supplements. Many people who believe they need to take a multivitamin supplement perhaps just aren't thinking about food in the right way. Broccoli is high in fibre, vitamin C, vitamin K, vitamin B9, iron, magnesium and potassium - and that is just one food. If I were to list all the nutritional benefits of avocado here, it would be a long and boring (but very healthy) list. These foods *are* multivitamins.

While supplements have their place, remember that food is about so much more than the nutrients you consume. It's about love, enjoyment and connection. You can't get that in a pill.

Alcohol

Drinking alcohol is one area where the correlation between lifestyle choices and risk of cancer is unequivocal. According to Cancer Research UK, alcohol can cause seven different types of cancer, with the evidence linking it to breast cancer particularly robust. According to CRUK stats, around 4,400 breast cancer cases each year are caused by drinking alcohol, and the risk increases even at low levels of drinking. So, no matter your starting point, the more you can cut down, the more you can reduce your risk.

'Alcohol is a carcinogen,' says Dr O'Riordan. 'We know it can cause cancer by itself, but also alcohol has no nutritional value – it's only metabolised to fat. And the more fat you have, the more oestrogen you make after the menopause, which increases your risk of breast cancer. So they suggest fewer than five units a week, but definitely not binge-drinking, so don't go out and have them all on a Saturday night.'

There are several ways in which alcohol causes cancer. It can damage cells and prevent cell repair. It can affect chemical signals, making cells more likely to divide. As Dr O'Riordan mentioned, there is also a theory that it affects women's hormone levels, increasing the amount of oestrogen in the body, which is then used by breast cancer cells as fuel for growth.

Interestingly, CRUK are keen to clarify that it is alcohol itself that causes damage, so it doesn't matter what type of alcohol you drink. This advice runs counter to the commonly held idea that a glass of red wine does you good, unlike, for example, a gin and tonic. Red wine has acquired something of a halo effect over the years, in light of research showing that the polyphenol resveratrol from the red grape skin could be good for your heart. Of course, you could just eat the grapes, but don't let me get in the way of your headline. Other research comparing people who have one small glass of red wine a day to teetotallers found that the wine-drinkers lived longer. But – and it's a big but – those studies are purely observational. So it might not be that the red wine is good for your heart, rather that the wine-drinkers made time each day to sit and enjoy dinner as a social occasion, improving collective wellbeing.

Also, people who don't drink at all might have existing health issues, which are the reason they don't drink in the first place. Or they may have replaced the function that alcohol might serve in their life (for example, socialising or managing negative emotions) with sugary or processed foods. Meanwhile, the one-small-red-wine-a-day people are eating a healthy Mediterranean diet of fresh veg, whole foods and good fats. It's pretty clear who is going to emerge from that situation healthier, and it's not because of the wine.

Anyway, alcohol causes cancer. That is well documented and not a controversial statement. But weirdly, the evidence is different when it comes to your risk of recurrence. 'Alcohol is an interesting one,' agrees Dr Nina Fuller-Shavel. 'It definitely significantly increases risk of primary breast cancer. In fact, there is no safe level of alcohol in terms of preventing primary breast cancer. But, in terms of recurrence risk, the data is not the same actually. Some studies even show a protective effect from moderate drinking. But most clinicians will say that it doesn't make sense why it would be protective for risk of recurrence. There must be something fishy going on in the way someone's run that particular study.'

Dr Fuller-Shavel also makes the point that drinking is socially acceptable, to the extent that people can often face resistance if they try to cut down. Also, it can become a habit that creeps into your daily life in quite a subtle way. 'When we hit perimenopause and menopause, we've often got older parents and young kids, and we're stressed out with work and it's not uncommon for a lot of women to put away half a bottle of wine at night,' she says. 'That significantly exceeds people's capacity, and it's often not noticeable because nobody gets drunk and nobody's out of control in any way. But actually, it all stacks up over time.'

Making it stick

At this point, you might be thinking: Yes, I know I need to eat the rainbow and drink less booze, but try telling that to my brain during after-work drinks on Friday nights, when I'm surrounded by cheap white wine and crisps. For some people, hearing the hard facts about the enormous health benefits of particular lifestyle changes is enough to get them to alter their behaviour. For others, however, having that information in their brains simply doesn't translate to the choices that they make in day-to-day life.

Back in 2017, in my pre-cancer life, I wrote a book called *Mindful Drinking*. It sprung from the idea that there exist lots of books about how to stop drinking, but many people don't want to stop altogether; they just want to be able to drink a bit less. What I learned about human behaviour change over the course of writing that book has affected every part of my life, in a positive way.

One of the key things that people fail to do when implementing lifestyle changes is to consider what kind of a person they are. For example, when it comes to healthy eating, some people's weakness is comfort food to cope with boredom or loneliness, and results in evening binge-eating in front of the television. For others, their trigger could be a people-pleasing tendency that requires them to eat every slice of cake they are offered and end up making their own so they can offer it in return.

I learned that my healthy-eating downfall was stress. When I worked in an office, I would generally have a healthy breakfast and lunch but, when it got to around 4 p.m. and I was a bit tired with deadlines suddenly feeling oppressive, I would scour the office for snacks. I worked in women's magazines and there always seemed to be cupcakes or doughnuts up for grabs in the afternoon. I'd tell myself that I just needed a hit of something sweet to get through the last few hours of the day, but would inevitably end up mindlessly stress-eating my way through a mountain of crap and then feeling quite sick on the way home.

Identifying your triggers, and understanding what you need and when, means that you can organise your life in a way that makes it easier to be healthy. It's about recognising and deconstructing your cravings, rather than trying to quash them. And this works for everything. If you've been dragging yourself to an after-work spin class that is nothing but a miserable experience, then could it be that you're a morning person and need to get your exercise in early? Or maybe the class setting is not for you, and something you can do on your own like running might be the answer?

So many people read about an eating plan or some other health-related strategy and try to incorporate it into their life without working out whether it's actually the right thing for them. And then they're annoyed with themselves for failing to stick with it.

For example, if you hate cooking, you're never going to enjoy whipping up nutritious meals from scratch. But convenience foods needn't be unhealthy; there are loads of great options available now and, if all else fails, chopped-up veg with hummus is my personal go-to meal when I'm on my own (I don't hate cooking for others, but can't be bothered to do it for myself – one of many reasons why having my family around is good for my health).

So cultivate self-awareness around each area of health, and think about what would work to help you make healthier choices in the relevant department.

Lots of people find accountability to be a huge driver of behaviour change so, if that sounds like you, arrange to meet a friend for that exercise class, or ask a colleague to check in with you to ensure you're eating a nutritious lunch every day.

Some people respond really well to a habit-tracking strategy of some description. This could take the form of an app like Dry Days, which allows you to tick off alcohol-free days in a rather satisfying way. Deliciously Ella's app, Feel Better, allows you to log the number of plant-based foods you've eaten, with an aim of having 30 different types a week. And the Oura ring monitors your sleep and movement, reminding you to go to bed early and get up from your desk to move around if you've been still for too long. However, some people find alerts from an app infuriating, and would never manage to keep on top of logging their food or drinks. If this is you, don't do it. Find another way that works for you.

Immunity

The power of the immune system is something that came up over and over again in my research, and I found it so interesting because I previously thought of it only in terms of fighting off colds and infections - not cancer. Nutritional scientist Toral Shah describes your immune system as being 'like a very fancy CCTV system', designed to spot and destroy cancer cells. A big part of the integrative nutrition for breast cancer courses she runs is about supporting your immunity through a diet rich in nutrients, anti-inflammatory ingredients and foods to support the gut microbiome.

The trouble is, explains Dr Liz O'Riordan, that cancer cells can evade the immune system's attempts to identify them. 'They have ways of sneaking past so they're not detected,' she says. 'The idea is that when you've got single cancer cells, the immune system's B-cells, T-cells and neutrophils will recognise them and pick them off. Immunotherapy is trying to change and strengthen the receptors on the immune cells, so they can detect cancer cells and pick them up. You can't make your B-cells suddenly much better at targeting cancer (with lifestyle), but you can strengthen your immune system overall. And how do you do that?'

Here she sighs a big sigh, and I know she's about to repeat

what we have said many times in this part of the book. 'You exercise, you eat well, you sleep well, you drink water, you avoid stress. All of those things just mean you're healthier. If you're rundown, doing 10-hour days back-to-back, not sleeping properly and getting McDonald's late at night . . . you'll be exhausted and have a migraine and then you'll get a chest infection because your body's saying you've done too much.' Which clearly doesn't put your immune system in the best position to function optimally.

As someone whose cancer was triple negative, I'm particularly interested in immune function. Soon after my diagnosis, I took part in an NHS-run nutrition course over Zoom, where they showed a graphic depicting how blood sugar spikes affect your hormones and turn healthy cells into cancer cells. When I asked if this effect was the same for TNBC tumours, the nutritionist running the course said no. She said that, while diet and lifestyle can hugely impact hormone receptor-driven cancers, they have no impact on TNBC. This was rather demoralising to hear at the time. I've been really interested to learn how important the immune system is in treating TNBC, and reducing risk of recurrence, since it feels like something I can effectively and proactively support.

'We're realising that the immune system is really highly important for triple negative,' says Dr Nina Fuller-Shavel. 'That's why we're now treating people up front with immunotherapy, because they can be quite immunogenic tumours but they're good at suppressing the immune system. So I would say that optimising someone's immune system is important for reducing their risk of recurrence. What I can't give you right now is a good interventional trial on it.' But, given her clinical experience and other available data, Dr Fuller-Shavel does assess and work on immune support and immunomodulation as a part of personalised integrative treatment. 'Even with people who have ongoing disease, actually it's much better controlled when we provide them with a good support,' she explains. 'So that means optimising vitamin D, making sure they have good nutrition to support the immune system, and ensuring inflammation is as low as possible.

She says that people are often discharged after cancer treatment showing lots of abnormal results in their blood tests. For example, a low neutrophil count or levels of nutrients such as iron or vitamin D. But, since treatment is over and the deficiency hasn't made the person seriously ill (yet), they just assume it will normalise and don't even tell the patient.

'I'm a scientist so I don't like assumptions,' says Dr Fuller-Shavel. 'My goal is not to just normalise those levels; it's to optimise a patient's life. I want to send people out feeling better than before they were diagnosed, and ensure the patient is not in the same terrain as they were when they got cancer. Many patients hear that the surgeon got all of the cancer out, so they don't change anything in their life and they recreate the same environment. But the definition of insanity is doing the same thing again, and expecting different results.'

Nutritional steps that you can take to support your immune system include metabolic control, which simply means keeping your blood sugar levels balanced, and good gut health. About 70 per cent of our immunity is in our gut, so diet is key for this. But please don't panic-buy probiotic supplements, as food generally has more bioavailability – that is, the nutrients in food are more easily absorbed and utilised by the body. We already know we should be eating a wide range of different-coloured vegetables and avoiding sugar, alcohol and processed foods, but you might not know that protein is essential for our immune systems to heal and build antibodies.

If you don't eat meat, it can be trickier to get 'complete proteins', i.e. foods that contain all nine amino acids, the building blocks of protein. Quinoa is one of the best plant-based complete proteins, and you can combine foods with different amino acids (for example, legumes like beans with grains such as rice).

Fibre is the other immunity-strengthening food group that is often overlooked and, again, it is found in many plant foods including fruit and veg, and nuts and beans. Also make sure you're getting enough B vitamins, found in eggs and fish.

And, apart from your diet, just look after yourself in general. 'If you are constantly having to fight coughs and colds because you're knackered, then your immune system is wearing out,' says Dr O'Riordan. 'Maybe every three months just take a moment to rebalance: Am I doing too much? How am I eating? Am I sleeping? What's my diet like? Reset the clock and start again. We all make mistakes. Just try to look after yourself.'

Stress Management

First, let's be clear about what stress is, because I'm aware that managing stress sounds like a flimsy nice-to-have rather than a biologically vital condition. You may have heard of the stress response, or 'fight or flight' response, which is when your body reacts to a stressful situation with tense muscles, quick breathing, sweating, gut issues and a racing heart. For thousands of years, this only really happened in response to physical danger. But now modern life has brought endless stressors, from reading about rapes and murders in the news, to the ongoing threat of wars and climate change, down to the relentless ping of work emails and the expectation of an immediate reaction to every work or personal crisis, no matter how small.

Unfortunately, the long-term effects of chronic stress on physical and psychological health are extremely wide-ranging. Repeated activation of the stress response takes an enormous toll on your body, impacting everything from your immunity to your blood pressure, causing brain changes that may contribute to anxiety, depression and addiction. Chronic stress also contributes to obesity, not only causing people to eat more (remember the stress eating I mentioned earlier?) but also by affecting sleep and hormone balance.

Meanwhile the relaxation response, or 'rest and digest', allows your body to calm down, regulating all of your physiological processes. As the name suggests, it lets you digest, but it also allows your brain and immune system to recover and heal.

This is all down to the autonomic nervous system, which has two components: the sympathetic nervous system, which you can think of as being like the accelerator pedal in a car – it triggers the 'fight or flight' response, providing the body with that nervous energy to respond to perceived dangers. And the parasympathetic nervous system, which is like the brake, promoting the 'rest and digest' response that calms the body down.

It's important to say that stress does not directly cause cancer. I say this because I know from experience that it can become a horrible vicious circle of feeling stressed about recurrence, and then panicking that your stress is increasing your chance of having recurrence, and then your stress is exacerbated and so on, and on, and on. Having said that, managing stress is a big part of looking after yourself, so can only help reduce your risk.

'Anecdotally, you see a lot of women who are very, very stressed who either get recurrences or get cancer,' says Dr Liz O'Riordan. 'Stress doesn't cause cancer, we can't blame it all on that. But women are good at taking on 50 things and juggling them. You need to look after yourself and think: Right, I'm exhausted. What can I stop? Can I just have a bath for half an hour? How can I recharge, to keep me as healthy as possible?'

There are certain times in life when acute stress is not only likely but a normal and expected reaction to events around you. A cancer diagnosis is clearly one of those times. It might hit you at diagnosis, during cancer treatment or later, after treatment. Long-term chronic stress may contribute to a range of health problems, including digestive disorders, headaches, sleep disorders, depression and anxiety, and other mental health problems. So, as much as we'd like to bury our heads in work, family stuff or a Netflix series and pretend it isn't happening, it's important to address it.

There are stress-management techniques that are designed to induce your body's relaxation response. The two most important are physical exercise (that old chestnut), and social support, so close ties with friends, family and your local community.

Beyond these are techniques that you can learn from a professional therapist or counsellor, such as CBT and PMR (progressive muscle relaxation). One common structured group stress-reduction programme studied in oncology in the US is called cognitive behavioural stress management (CBSM).

There are also many apps with guided meditations and breathing exercises. Basically, it's anything that helps to calm your body, encourage your shoulders to drop, enable you to breathe deeply and deal with your stress in a healthy way. You might need to try out a few techniques before landing on the one that works for you.

The brain is built to keep you alive, which means it's wired to scan your environment constantly for everything that could go wrong, or whatever might bring you harm. This also means that brains have a tendency to focus on the negative over the positive, which is known as 'negativity bias'. But your brain being biased doesn't mean you have to be. By regularly choosing to focus on the positive in a situation, or seeking out the positive things in your environment (such as the people you love, the music you enjoy, and making an effort to derive pleasure from simple things like a sunny day), you can help train your brain to be less reactive to negative circumstances.

And don't underestimate the power of human touch. A hug, affectionate touch or even a bit of self-massage encourages the release of oxytocin, which negates the effects of cortisol, the stress hormone that can weaken the immune system and deplete your white blood cells.

If you have to do a task that you know is going to stress you out, then there are ways you can trick your brain into feeling a bit more relaxed. Fragrance such as lavender and citrus is good for soothing your nervous system, as is relaxing music. Do everything you can to make the experience less stressful, and it'll pay off in every part of your life, from your sleep to your immunity.

The important thing to remember about managing stress is that it's not about eliminating it. That would be impossible. Every single one of us, to a greater or lesser degree, has stressors around us all the time. And sometimes they can be positive, giving us the push we need to have a tricky conversation or meet a deadline. But constant stress can be detrimental to your mental health, your nervous system and, in turn, your immunity. So it's about finding techniques to help you cope with it.

Life is obviously too short to stew over pointless disagreements, or tolerate spending any more time than you absolutely have to with toxic people. If you have a difficult person in your life, be that at work, in your wider friendship group or – worst of all – in your family, then you won't necessarily be able to avoid them completely. Instead, think of them as a child. I've used this technique when dealing with high-maintenance people and it's incredibly useful. If you saw a tantrum-ing four-year-old, you wouldn't take it personally. You would assume they're probably tired or hangry, and would respond with calm acknowledgement until they simmered down. Usually a difficult person has had a difficult time in life, so approach the situation with compassion, understanding that the issue is with them, not with you. You can't control other people's actions, but you can control the way in which you respond to them, which can usually make a huge difference.

Remember: there will never be a point where you've cracked it, and stressful situations are no longer an issue. Stress is part of life, so this is a lifelong practice.

Breathwork

Breathing is one of the quickest and most effective tools at your disposal for managing stress and anxiety. It feels insultingly obvious to state how vital oxygen is for the healthy functioning of many of the body's systems (including immunity), because it's an automatic process. But you only have to look at those tech bros in Silicon Valley who are using breathwork to biohack their cognitive function, manage stress and increase energy to see how powerful it can be.

The process of writing this book actually provided me with a pertinent example of the importance of slow, steady breathing. While researching the subject of breast cancer recurrence and metastasis to write the chapter on secondary breast cancer, I felt sick and dizzy, with a racing heart. It was only when I closed my eyes to take a moment that I realised I was holding my breath. I realised how our bodies can react to uncomfortable feelings in a very visceral way. The deep fear of what I was learning about had caused me to stop breathing, in turn causing distressing physical symptoms. It was eye-opening.

Reminding yourself to breathe slowly and deeply is something that you can do right now. It can help you refocus, and make smarter decisions about how you spend your time and emotional energy. Breathwork is also said to improve cellular renewal and lymphatic flow, so it's even more vital for anyone with a cancer diagnosis. But – and I understand that I am not alone in this – I often find that when I attempt to focus on my breath, I seem to totally forget how to breathe and become actually quite breathless.

'That is very normal,' assures Stuart Sandeman, breathwork coach and author of *Breathe In, Breathe Out*. 'Often when I ask people to close their eyes and be aware of their breath, not trying to change it in any way, they panic, like, "Argh, how am I breathing right now?!"' Why does this happen? 'It's because you've brought awareness to it, which brings us to a space that we don't often connect to with a busy mind. It can feel almost claustrophobic.'

Claustrophobic is exactly how I feel when I try to slow my breath. Stuart explains that this can trigger an anxious brain to panic that you're not breathing enough. So, as I'm trying to do a relaxing slow out-breath, my brain is screaming: 'Take a freakin' breath in!'

'Take baby steps,' advises Stuart. 'Go into it slowly, reminding yourself that you can take a breath at any point. That should override that feeling. Because if your brain senses any threat, either externally in our environment or internally through our thoughts, it will trigger faster breathing and shorter, shallow breaths into our chest.'

The trouble is, we can get stuck in this fast-breathing pattern, which in turn rings the alarm bell to the brain, like a loop of stress. So it's about persevering with slow, deep breaths, while reminding your brain that – here and now – you are safe.

Stuart's advice for that spiralling 4 a.m. anxiety, or the general sense of overwhelm with which we're all familiar, is a technique called Recognise, Breathe, Reframe. 'Try to objectively look at a situation, with a bird's eye view, and acknowledge how you're feeling,' he says. 'It's really important not to sweep it under the carpet because we just end up trapping it and holding on to it.'

So think about how you're feeling and why you're feeling that way, then breathe in deeply to your belly and make a humming sound for as long as you can while breathing out. Do that for 90 seconds, then reframe your thoughts. That might mean reminding yourself there is a greater chance that the cancer won't come back, and you're doing all you can to reduce your risk. After taking the time to breathe it out, other ideas might come to you. It might be: I need to find more ways to relax my body, which calms my mind. Maybe I'll go to yoga tomorrow.

Cold-water swimming

Cold-water immersion has been shown to have many physical and mental health benefits, and adding swimming into the mix gives you a full-body workout. After all, cold water has long been considered an excellent natural pain reliever, but we now know that it can also reduce inflammation and kick-start the immune system, strengthening your defences against the onslaught of cancer treatment.

Other benefits in terms of breast cancer are said to include helping your liver cope with regulating hot flushes during a perimenopausal moment, and encouraging blood flow to protect your vital organs, which is great for your circulation if you do it regularly.

It appears that regularity is key. The initial cold shock activates the stress response but, after a few chilly dips, your body adapts and actually learns to deal with stress better. You might not imagine that the benefits transfer to emotional stress, but it seems they do, in a process called cross-adaptation. It's a mood-boosting activity, with euphoric feelings reported after a cold-water dip, which scientists put down to a flood of endorphins in response to the shock of the temperature. If you swim outside, with others, then there are also the additional psychological benefits of spending time in nature and being part of a community.

Even after researching and writing about the extraordinary benefits of cold-water swimming, will I do it? No. This is a perfect example of my regular refrain that you have to find what works for you, because everybody's different. And cold water on my body does not work for me. Ask anybody who has ever stepped outside a building with me between November and March: I hate being cold. The good news for me, and those who feel the way I do about cold water, is that swimming in any temperature is excellent after breast cancer treatment. Not only is it a good low-impact full-body exercise, but also the pressure of the water is an in-built lymphatic massage.

Having read so much about the benefits of cold water, I have tried it. I've tried switching my shower to cold in the morning, and I've tried getting into a cold plunge pool in a spa, but I simply can't bear it. I have made peace with the fact that I was born to be warm. Now I listen to the cold-water converts enthusing about breaking the ice to swim in the lido, and I simply smile and say comedian Amy Poehler's favourite phrase: 'Good for you, not for me.'

Step back from the news cycle

Yes, I know it's important to be informed, and you might even have a job that requires you to keep on top of the news (mine used to, and arguably still does to an extent), but you don't have to consume news stories quite so relentlessly.

I once wore an HRV (or heart rate variability) tracker for 24 hours to monitor my activity, stress levels and fatigue. When I sat down with a doctor to go through my results, I made an interesting discovery

'What was happening at 1.30 p.m.?' asked the doctor, pointing to a point on the chart where my stress levels skyrocketed. I told her I was eating lunch.

'Did you hate your lunch?'

'No, it was delicious.'

'Were you doing anything else?'

'Umm . . . I was reading the paper?'

'Ah-ha!'

She went on to explain that because we're so accustomed to it, our brain doesn't even acknowledge the stress we feel when reading a series of grim news stories. But our body knows, and our nervous system was simply not designed to hear about a war, a natural disaster and a disturbing investigation into what children are watching on YouTube – all in the 20 minutes that it takes to eat your lunch.

So think about changing the way in which you consume news. If you don't need to know every event of the day as it happens, then try not scrolling through news websites during the week. Perhaps the Sunday papers can be a time when you catch up on everything – the bleak news tempered by the joy of style and culture supplements.

Edit who you follow on social media, so you're not seeing depressing headlines appearing in amongst updates from friends and family. If a big news story happens, believe me, you'll hear about it. You will only be missing out on things you don't need to know about anyway. If you do feel that you need to keep on top of the news every day, then the one change I ask you to make is, don't read or watch it last thing at night. Which brings me to the next point...

Sleep

When it comes to cancer, and also general good health, sleep is often overlooked in favour of more active interventions like nutrition and movement.

'Both sleep and stress are the underrated elements here, the underdogs,' says Dr Nina Fuller-Shavel. 'And not enough is made of that because actually the evidence is pretty strong.' The trouble is, so many people have come to accept being constantly stressed and sleeping badly as part of life, they don't take addressing those issues seriously. 'But if we accept general crappiness, we are going to get crappiness back,' insists Dr Fuller-Shavel. 'I am very hot on sleep and stress with patients who have had a primary diagnosis, because it does appear to be associated with survival, and it does appear to be associated with the risk of recurrence. We know association is not causation. However, given the additional evidence on the influence of sleep and chronic stress on immune, metabolic and mental health, it is important to pay attention. I don't remember any of my doctors ever asking me about sleep when I had breast cancer. I always ask people about it, but I'm probably one of the only doctors who does.'

When it comes to emotional wellbeing, the importance of sleep cannot be overstated. Insufficient sleep can leave you emotionally exhausted, and more prone to irritability and stress. Chronic insomnia may increase the risk of a mood disorder like anxiety or depression. And if you are postmenopausal, or cancer treatment has stopped your periods, then the symptoms of that – such as mood swings and difficulty concentrating or remembering things – can be hugely exacerbated by a lack of sleep.

A study from the University of Bern mapped the activity of neurons during rapid eye movement sleep (REM) and found that the sleeping brain reinforces positive emotions and weakens negative ones – which is why an argument never seems as bad once you've slept on it.

Not only have studies shown that night-shift nurses have higher rates of colorectal and breast cancer, those data are now so good that the World Health Organization has listed night-shift work as a probable carcinogen.

What's the answer if you just can't sleep? Well, it feels easy to reach for a sleeping pill, but the ones that are often prescribed during cancer treatment, such as zopiclone or zolpidem, are highly addictive and don't actually deliver good-quality sleep. Of course, they are good for knocking you out in an emergency, and I certainly used them when I was wired on steroids or struggling with post-surgical pain. But studies have shown that they don't provide proper, restorative sleep, so are not a long-term solution.

You will probably have heard of using sleep hygiene techniques as a way to encourage natural, deep sleep. Don't dismiss them, even if you think that you already sleep well, because they can really improve the quality of your sleep, as well as how well you stay asleep. They include things like limiting caffeine, sticking to a regular schedule of when you get up and go to bed, ensuring your bedroom is dark, cool and free of electronic devices, and implementing some kind of pre-bedtime wind-down routine, which could be having a bath, doing some gentle stretches or breathing exercises, or just reading a book.

Things to avoid for a couple of hours before bed include eating a heavy meal, looking at screens, and drinking alcohol (although it may knock you out initially, you're likely to wake in the night with your heart racing).

What you do earlier in the day also affects your sleep. Getting outside as early as you can after sunrise every day will get some natural light on your skin, regulating your melatonin levels by telling your body it's morning time. This is also a good idea in terms of boosting your vitamin D. You might not feel like it in winter, but that's when it's even more important. So, if you see the sun peeping out from behind a cloud on a cold day – go outside as soon as you can and get that precious light on your face.

As you can see, although I have broken up these elements of good health, they are all intertwined. If you have a poor night's sleep, you are more likely to overeat and reach for highly processed convenience foods. You're less likely to find the energy to exercise, or the time to meditate. Therefore you sleep badly again the next night, and the next day is even worse. It's a vicious circle, but one that can be broken by implementing lifestyle changes. As always, you have to look at the big picture, because all the sleep hygiene techniques in the world won't help if you're not eating well, moving your body and managing stress. These things will have a huge positive impact on your sleep, and on every part of your physical and emotional wellbeing.

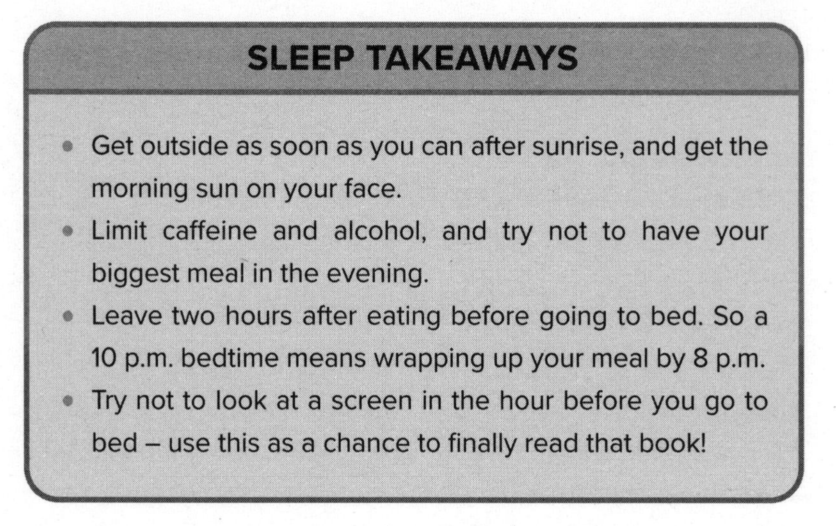

SLEEP TAKEAWAYS

- Get outside as soon as you can after sunrise, and get the morning sun on your face.
- Limit caffeine and alcohol, and try not to have your biggest meal in the evening.
- Leave two hours after eating before going to bed. So a 10 p.m. bedtime means wrapping up your meal by 8 p.m.
- Try not to look at a screen in the hour before you go to bed – use this as a chance to finally read that book!

Spirituality

I was raised in a home with no religious faith, went to a secular school, and have never believed in any kind of god. It was never something that bothered me. In fact, I was kind of proud to be a rational person who put their trust in science, not in some higher power. But over the years, I've increasingly started to wish that I did.

It's often reported that people who have a structured faith are happier, healthier and live longer. And I've always assumed that this is down to the things that usually come as part of the package of having religious beliefs: gratitude, charity, forgiveness and a sense of community. There is also research to show the benefits of the meditative contemplation of prayer, and even singing as part of a group. Singing stimulates your vagus nerve, which interacts with your heart, lungs and digestive tract, relaxing your breathing, heart rate and gut. It's a powerful stress-buster that does wonders for your immune system.

During Dan Buettner's pioneering work into the Blue Zones, parts of the world in which people live healthier lives for longer, he whittled down their longevity to nine factors. Among the things you might expect, such as eating well (lots of veg, fibre, polyphenols, you know the drill by now), moving their bodies, having a good sense of community ... all but five of the 263 centenarians his team interviewed belonged to some kind of faith-based community. Denomination didn't seem to matter. Whatever your religion, it seems that attending faith-based services four times a month will add between four and 14 years on to your life expectancy.

Kelly Turner found a similar thing when she was researching her book, *Radical Remission: Surviving Cancer Against All Odds*. You might have heard stories of people given a terminal cancer diagnosis who then miraculously become cancer-free, often with minimal conventional interventions. She tracked down as many of these medical anomalies as she could and asked them what they did: what changes they made, what they thought made their cancers spontaneously shrink. As a researcher and PhD doctor, she is the first to caveat their stories with the fact that they're anecdotal and there is little clinical evidence behind their astonishing recoveries. But these people have been dismissed by medical studies because they don't fit in with what is supposed to happen when you have stage four cancer. She reasons that breakthroughs have been made in the past after studying anomalies, so it's worth investigating.

Perhaps predictably, perhaps reassuringly, lots of what these people did is what we have already covered here: having good social connections, taking control of your health and eating the rainbow (although she recommends giving up dairy, which is not evidence-based and, as a cheese-lover, I don't think I could). But one of the key findings is that most of the people with spontaneous remission had a deep spiritual connection.

So is being an atheist bad for my health? Actually, the word atheist suggests a level of certainty that there is no higher power out there and who can actually know that for sure?

I have had the occasional experience when I thought maybe there is, or might be, something bigger than us.

Shortly after my cancer treatment finished, I was sent to review a luxury medical spa called Lanserhof in Germany for a newspaper feature (I know, it's a tough job). Lanserhof's ethos is all about helping you 'live better for longer', and I arrived there with my spirit broken. My fear of recurrence was so all-encompassing that I was having phantom symptoms, including back and neck pain, every day. A brilliantly brisk and efficient doctor excavated my fears with direct questions about my experience of cancer treatment, which left me an emotional wreck in her pristine white clinic. She told me I needed to have my energy healed, got me to lie on the treatment table and then performed what felt like something of an exorcism. She lit what she called 'fire sticks' and waved them around as I felt warm vibrations flowing through me. Then it honestly felt as though my mind floated up out of my body. Afterwards I felt so much better, lighter, cleansed. I thanked her and she replied, 'It wasn't me,' gesturing to the sky. Having been fully on board with the process moments earlier, her allusion to God suddenly made me doubt it.

So, yes, now I do kind of wish I had a religious faith. If you have one, albeit lapsed, then I would say that having cancer is certainly the time to lean into it, if that feels comfortable for you. I understand that some people have had negative, or even traumatic, experiences as a result of acts of oppression or abuses of power in the name of religion. I wouldn't recommend anyone return to a faith that has not served them well in the past. But if you've let elements of the faith into which you were born slide over the years, then this could be a good time to resurrect them, as the benefits are well documented.

If, like me, you don't have a religious faith, there are ways in which it's possible to capture some of the magic of belief in a higher power. I used to be more cynical about such things but, as time goes on, I think I am starting to believe in the concept of energy, and that we're all connected.

Fearne Cotton's book, *Bigger Than Us*, is a brilliantly matter-of-fact investigation into the ways that we can find a spiritual connection through simple practices such as yoga, meditation, energy therapies and connection. The word 'God' is never mentioned in the book. Instead, it's about everyday things we can do to, as she says, 'find meaning in a messy world'. It's this idea of meaning that is so powerful, because if we feel that life is meaningless then what do we have to live for?

Community

One way to incorporate the benefits of organised religion into your life is by fostering a sense of community. Connection with other people is one of the best things you can do for your health, because our nervous system is constantly searching for assurance that we're safe, and that so often comes through conversation. Like food and shelter, a sense of belonging is a basic human need. And, despite how loving and supportive your family or partner might be, one person cannot fulfil all of your emotional needs, so it's important to make an effort to maintain your social circle.

People often believe that friendships and strong relationships come naturally. Films and television shows portray large, warm, supportive friendship groups, which seem to form organically without anyone working on it. In reality of course, if you don't consciously decide to make an effort to check in with your friends when they're going through a tough time, or occasionally be the one to arrange the catch-up dinners, then you'll find your social circle starts to shrink pretty quickly.

Looser social connections are also surprisingly important; it's a case of chatting to the person that makes your coffee as you're dashing for the train, or having a chat with the postman about the weather. This is something that we often take for granted, but we lost many of these opportunities during the Covid pandemic. Unplanned connections are so vital. Be a person that other people want to be around. Learn to affirm and appreciate other people. And be aware that how you think and feel rubs off on others. This is why some people create a sense of anxiety, just by being around them.

As social creatures, the energy exchange that occurs during human interaction nourishes us and has numerous health benefits, including immune system support. Loneliness has been shown to be as bad for your health as smoking. The statistics about that should be a wake-up call for anyone who still believes that emotional and physical wellbeing are not intrinsically connected. In his book, *When the Body Says No*, Gabor Maté explains that he doesn't even like the term 'connected' as that implies two separate entities, and they are one. So think about the traditions and practices you can fit into your life, inspired by religious faiths.

RITUALS FOR THE NON-RELIGIOUS

Gratitude Making lists of things for which you are grateful is one of the best-known and often-quoted ways to feel happier.

Song Studies have shown that singing is an effective mood-booster and stress-reliever, even if carried out alone. Do it as part of a group to reap the further benefits of connection and community. Perhaps join a choir or attend more live music events.

Prayer Could your version of praying take the form of meditation, a breathing practice, yoga, or simply taking time to focus on nothing but stroking your cat?

Charity If you can, donate to a local food bank, or consider running 10k to raise money for a good cause. Check out the resources section for charities who are providing vital support for people with cancer.

Ritual You don't have to burn sage during the full moon (although you can if you want to!). A simple ritual could be journaling or just lighting a candle while you have a bath.

You don't have to worry that you're not 'doing it right', or fear that you're being glib about actual religion. It's about what feels right for you, and what gives you that greater sense of meaning. You could even take something that you already do and enjoy, and find a way to focus purely on it, really appreciating the headspace that it provides. In the spirit of this, a friend once told me that 'running is my church'. Find your own way, with your own rituals, in your own tradition.

The Future of Breast Cancer Treatment

Breast cancer treatment has come on leaps and bounds in the last few decades, and continues to develop at an astonishing rate. The treatment I had for primary triple negative breast cancer (TNBC) included an adjuvant chemotherapy drug called capecitabine, which was not being widely used until just a few years ago.

Meanwhile, Trodelvy is a comparatively new drug which can extend the lives of women with metastatic TNBC. It received a lot of attention in 2022, after it was initially rejected by NICE for being too expensive for use within the NHS. Over the next three months, a campaign led by Breast Cancer Now garnered an unprecedented amount of attention, with 215,000 people signing a petition and 27 cross-party parliamentarians adding their names to an open letter to the drug company Gilead, asking them to make the drug available to those who need it. In July 2022, Trodelvy's provisional rejection was reversed and it was approved by NICE for routine use on the NHS.

Further research that same year showed the drug Enhertu

– which was already being used on the NHS to treat some women with HER2 metastatic breast cancer – can benefit many more women whose tumour cells contain lower levels of the HER2 protein.

Due to the speed at which new drugs are coming to market, there will inevitably be situations where people find themselves missing out on a wonder drug because it was only available after they were treated. This is exactly what happened to me in 2021.

After having been through chemotherapy, mastectomy surgery and radiotherapy, I was writing an article for the *Sunday Times* about the future of cancer treatment, for which I interviewed several experts. Imagine my initial excitement and then dismay as one of them – Professor Peter Schmid, who features in this book – told me about an immunotherapy drug that had been found to reduce the risk of recurrence by 40 per cent in patients with primary TNBC. Professor Schmid enthused about the amazing results he had seen in his private patients that year.

When I told him that I had just been treated for TNBC and had never even heard of, let alone been offered, this drug, he paused. Then he explained how new drugs often get approved more quickly by the FDA (Food and Drug Administration) in the US than they do by NICE in the UK. He said that private clinics can use these new drugs, based on American approval, but they are not available to NHS patients until they are approved by NICE. I happened to have been treated during the window that the drug – called pembrolizumab – was being used in the US and in private clinics in the UK, but not on the NHS.

A reduction in the rate of recurrence by 40 per cent is no small matter, particularly with TNBC, which comes with a higher rate of recurrence anyway. I asked if I could have it as an adjuvant treatment if I went private right away, but he explained it must be given with chemotherapy pre-surgery, when the tumour is still present. Since then, pembrolizumab has been approved for treatment of primary TNBC patients within the NHS.

I was initially so angry and frustrated that no one had told me. Since I didn't have health insurance, I'm not sure how I thought I was going to pay for it (and it would have cost upwards of £100,000, since you'd have to pay for private chemo at the same time), but that was beside the point. It would never have crossed my mind to ask if my treatment would be different had I had private healthcare, and I was annoyed that no one told me it was an option . . . until it wasn't.

Professor Schmid tells me he has had situations where patients have come to see him seeking immunotherapy and often, by the time they hear of it, they have had surgery so it's too late. It's one of the reasons why he's passionate about patients being given all of the information up front, and taking time to be sure about which option is best for them.

I obviously can't dwell on treatments that I didn't receive simply because I didn't pay for private healthcare, or was diagnosed 18 months too early to have it on the NHS. Okay, I did dwell on it rather furiously for a while. But now I have come to terms with that being the nature of the beast.

One key revelation over the last decade in breast cancer care has been the increased understanding that there are many more variables between different types of breast cancer than first thought, and the future will see a much more personalised approach.

Dr Niamh Buckley and Professor Helen McCarthy are currently leading a research team at Queen's University

Belfast, looking into treatment for TNBC tumours. The biggest change in cancer research over the last few years, Dr Buckley tells me, is an understanding of the role of the immune system (*see page 295*).

'The thing with the immune system is it can be a friend or a foe,' she explains. 'Potential cancers are occurring in our bodies every day, and our immune system is set up to recognise that a mistake has happened, and clear it out. But cancer will keep trying little things to hide from the immune system. Either it removes things from its surface so the immune system can't see it, or else it will disable the ability of the immune system to fight it. But [cancer cells] can also trick the immune system into actually working for them,' she continues. 'They harness the inflammation that the immune system uses when a wound is healing, when you actually want to grow lots of cells. And that's how immunotherapy treatments work: either by trying to stop the immune system from helping out the cancer, or by being able to reactivate the positive sides of the immune system. The other advantage of this is that if we can get the immune system working well, we know it has a memory. So it has the potential then to recognise your cancer if it recurs, and get rid of it.'

Dr Buckley and her team are working specifically on triple negative breast cancer because it has fewer targeted treatments available. We already know that TNBC is defined by not having any of the three targets most commonly present in breast cancer: ER+, PR+ and HER2. 'So it's not really one disease, it's lots of different diseases,' explains Dr Buckley. 'Some of the research over the last few years would say that there are six subgroups of triple negative, some will say there are 10. And what we're trying to do is find out how we can better understand the biology within its subgroups. We want to make sure that when a patient presents, we can say, you have *this type* of triple negative breast cancer. But that's going to take time, and it will mean that some drugs will only work for very few people. And cynics will say that drug companies love to develop drugs that they can give to everybody, because then they make more money,' she adds, with a raised eyebrow. 'Maybe that is a factor, but also it's harder to go through the clinical testing stages when you can only involve people with a very specific type of cancer. So it's just harder and probably slower. But that's where we need to go: where you're treating almost everybody as an individual, or at least as a subgroup.'

The treatment that the research team at Queen's University Belfast are working on is a vaccine that will target p53, a gene that appears in high levels in 80–90 per cent of triple negative tumours. 'We were working on this before Covid but, since the mRNA vaccine revolution, it's made it a lot easier for people to see how it can work,' she says. 'What we're hoping to do with the vaccine is to train the immune system to go after cells with those high levels of p53. We want the treatment to be as cancer-specific as we can. Because chemotherapy may kill cancer cells, but it kills lots of other cells as well. It's really tough.'

The idea of a vaccine that can prevent cancer might sound like a wildly futuristic concept but, actually, vaccines for cancer already exist. Human papillomavirus (HPV) vaccines, which are now given to all 12- to 13-year-olds in the UK, prevent cervical cancer by targeting the HPV strains that trigger tumour growths. The dream would be to train the body to recognise tumour cells, which is what the team at Queen's hope to do.

It's incredibly promising research and, while it will take time and fine-tuning, it could dramatically improve outcomes for women diagnosed with TNBC. Initially it will be a treatment rather than a preventative vaccine, but Dr Buckley says she could see it being used in a preventative capacity at some point in the future. Although probably only for people who are at high risk, with a family history of breast cancer.

Meanwhile, over in Ohio, the Cleveland Clinic is currently running trials on a vaccine that could prevent recurrence in women who have been treated for primary TNBC. And at Penn Medicine in Philadelphia, scientists are testing a vaccine that would train a group of immune cells in the body known as T-cells to identify and destroy cancer cells. The trial will, of course, take years to come to fruition, but it's reassuring that progress is being made.

Another big step forward in the future of cancer treatment is the development of 'liquid biopsies', whereby cancer can be diagnosed with a simple blood test. Dr Buckley says it's also something they've been looking at, as have cancer researchers all over the world. 'Where it will first come into play is in monitoring treatment response and looking for disease recurrence,' she says. 'But eventually it could move into early diagnosis screening.' The trouble, at the moment, is that these tests have not been as precise or as accurate as they need to be in order to become widely used. 'But there have been amazing trials run all over the world,' she adds. 'With melanoma, they've been able to do a blood test and actually see the cancer emerging before we can clinically detect it.'

This is exciting because early diagnosis is one of the most important elements in successful cancer treatment. And, as more of this new research gets tested in trials and licensed for use, breast cancer in the future will increasingly be about prevention and survivorship.

Surgical progress is also happening at a mind-boggling speed. For instance, DIEP flap surgery wasn't available until the 1990s, and wasn't widely used until recently. Now, surgical advances may present a breakthrough for women at risk of lymphoedema. A new technique called LYMPHA (Lymphatic Microsurgical Preventive Healing Approach) involves draining blocked lymphatic vessels by surgically creating a shunt between a lymphatic channel and a blood vessel. Oncoplastic breast surgeon Miss Georgette Oni tells me that, while it's an exciting development, it's far from being widely rolled out. 'I know they do quite a lot of it in the States, and I think there was a case that was done in London,' she says, 'but it's very fiddly, tricky and time-consuming. It would add quite a bit of time to the operation. I'm not aware of any long-term studies on it yet but, as more research is done in that area, it will become slicker, faster surgery. Ultimately, what they're looking at now is: can we avoid doing that clearance altogether?'

That's right. Rather than erring on the side of caution in terms of removing several (or in many cases, all) of the lymph nodes, there is a hope that in the future they will be able to identify patients whose chemotherapy has been so effective that all of the lymph nodes are cancer-free. This is something that they can't yet tell without removing them. But these kinds of advances could prevent many patients from having to have such aggressive surgery.

Miss Oni also tells me that there is much excitement about robotics and artificial intelligence being used in surgery, but it's still in the early stages – robots doing surgical procedures may be more precise but 'it just takes hours'.

On top of the scientific breakthroughs being made in research labs around the world, the shape of how cancer treatment will look in the future is changing for the better. Social media, other online resources, and even publications like this book are helping people to realise that there is so much they can do to support themselves through treatment and beyond. And more doctors and clinicians are upskilling themselves to acknowledge and support cancer patients' physical and psychological needs. It's reassuring to think that these advances will hugely benefit our daughters' and granddaughters' generations, and it makes me really optimistic about the future.

Summary

I'm aware that, over the course of this book, I have covered a lot of ground. The last thing I want is for you to feel overwhelmed. If you're reading this, the chances are you're dealing with your own diagnosis, so I don't want you to put pressure on yourself that – on top of everything – you now have a lot of new rules to follow. Think of this as a toolbox, there if you need it, for dipping in and out.

If I were to tie together the key threads of what I've learned over the course of writing this section, it would be that the simplest changes have the biggest impact. What you do every day matters more than what you do once in a while. So, when making lifestyle changes, make them small and doable.

Really simple steps are the best way to rebuild yourself after cancer treatment: your body *and* your mind. Resilience isn't learned through a corporate training session, or even through a book like this. It comes from experience, and a sense of togetherness that is fostered through a community, whatever that means to you.

You don't need to...	Instead, you might...
Spend a lot of money on supplements or goji berries.	Think of ways to add different-coloured veg to your diet.
Sweat it out in the gym if you hate it.	Have a 10-minute walk after lunch, do some squats while waiting for the kettle to boil.
Sacrifice your social life and go to bed at 9.30 p.m. every night.	Set up a sleep schedule on your phone, to avoid looking at screens after a certain time.
Never have sugar or alcohol ever again.	Buy the best quality you can afford and really enjoy it, while focusing on healthy choices most of the time.
Become a yoga guru who is calm and serene at all times.	Find a room and focus on your breath for five minutes when you feel overwhelmed.

There is a lot of talk in the cancer community about enjoying every moment of life post-treatment – living with constant gratitude and endlessly seizing the day. While this sounds great on paper (or on Instagram), it can make people feel as though they're failing because they're not fully appreciating every single minute.

Feeling under pressure to enjoy life is clearly counterproductive to actually enjoying it. Even a person who appears to have it all sussed out in terms of making healthy choices and having fulfilling relationships, will miss a train or stub a toe. And, beyond daily annoyances, all of us will have to deal with big life changes like personal or work-related rejections, or unforeseen disasters, or grief. Being relentlessly happy is an impossible goal. Not only is it not realistic, it's also undesirable. You can't have life's highs without the lows, after all. That's what life is.

Focus on increasing opportunities for meaningful social interactions and purposeful work. Remember there will never be a point where you feel that you've got it completely sussed so, as much of a cliché as this might be, try to appreciate the journey rather than longing for the destination. Actress Carrie Fisher used to talk about the meal and the bill. You know the bill is coming, she would say, so make sure that you enjoy the meal.

And when trying to instigate positive lifestyle changes, remember that life can often get in the way, and you have to allow it to ebb and flow. If you have small children who are up in the night, you're not going to get as much sleep as you'd like. If you have a big work project on that's taking up all of your time, socialising might be on the back burner for a while. If you're having a particularly sociable time, you're unlikely to be eating as healthily as you might normally. Don't let this stress you out; just accept it as part of life. You may be able to make healthy choices in every part of your life at various times, but probably not all at the same time. You're a human being, not a robot.

So was breast cancer 'the best thing that ever happened to me', as someone once told me it could be? Well, no. Cancer is a horrific disease, treatment is gruelling and traumatic, and managing anxiety about recurrence is an ongoing process. If I could wave a magic wand and not have had breast cancer, then I would absolutely do that.

But that's not to say that there haven't been positives to come out of the experience. Assuming the cancer doesn't come back (and I think we all have to try and live by that assumption), then I've certainly reduced my risk of many other chronic conditions, from heart disease to strokes, simply by making a few lifestyle changes. I've disavowed myself of the misconception that eating healthily means eliminating entire food groups, or being fit means trekking to the gym every day.

If reading this book has made you think that I'm some kind of paragon of virtue who always makes healthy choices, then I wish you could see the mountain of Tony's Chocolonely and enormous vat of coffee that I consumed while writing it. Life isn't about making perfect choices one hundred per cent of the time. It's about doing your best most of the time, and enjoying those moments when you've let it all go.

Since that bleak day in January 2021, when I knew life would never be the same again, I've been on a mission to future-proof my body, but in a realistic way. And I really hope that what I've learned is useful, reassuring and galvanising for you too. I hope I've inspired you to be bold about looking at your life and eliminating the things that no longer serve you, making more room for the things that bring joy.

If you take only one thing from this book, I want it to be that if you're feeling overwhelmed and like you're not coping, that is completely normal. Please don't feel like you're failing as a mother, a friend, a daughter, a wife, a human being. However you are feeling, it's a completely understandable reaction to what you're going or have been through. So cut yourself some slack. Treat yourself as you would a small child, with lots of rest, love, patience and understanding.

Yes, you want to make healthy choices to feel better and improve your chances of longevity. But it can be easy to get caught up in striving to over-analyse and optimise your health and happiness. Instead, live well by rejecting perfection.

You have come face to face with your own mortality and,

perhaps for the first time, you've thought deeply about what might happen when you die. This has been difficult and painful, but it's given you a chance to think about what you want to do with your life, and what you want to leave behind. Now you can make decisions about how you spend your time with clarity and intention, with your core values at the forefront of your mind. Because a breast cancer diagnosis might mean the end of your carefree former self, but it can also be the start of a life lived more fully.

References

1 Prue Cormie, 'Every cancer patient should be prescribed exercise medicine', theconversation.com, 6 May 2018

2 Rachel Grumman Bender, 'Kathy Bates on surviving cancer twice: "When you see what you're afraid of, you can face it"', yahoo.com, 6 March 2019

3 'Feminist Gloria Steinem Finds Herself Free Of The "Demands Of Gender"', Fresh Air / npr.org, 26 August 2016

4 Joan Baez on action, www.spiritualityhealth.com

5 'Medicinal mushrooms in cancer treatment', cancerres-earch.org, 4 November 2022

Resources

Action Cancer, the major cancer information and support charity in Northern Ireland, offers one-to-one counselling for free: 028 9080 3344, info@actioncancer.org

After Breast Cancer Diagnosis advocacy and information: ABCDiagnosis.co.uk

Beauty Despite Cancer by Jennifer Young is great for skincare during treatment: beautydespitecancer.com

Big Strong Lasses weight training for beginners online classes are run by Carolyn Garritt. For more details visit her website: www.oomph.london

Breast Cancer Now helpline to speak to an experienced breast care nurse: 0808 800 6000, breastcancernow.org

Cancer Rehab PT is a YouTube channel with videos showing how to exercise safely after surgery, and how to do lymphatic massage correctly: youtube.com/cancerrehabpt

Cancer Research UK has an extremely useful website, as well as a nurse freephone helpline: 0808 800 4040. cancerresearchuk.org

The C-List beauty platform for anyone going through cancer treatment: the-c-list.com

Flat Friends guide for living without reconstruction: flatfriends.org.uk

Future Dreams provides practical, emotional and psychological support through in-person or online events: futuredreams.org.uk

Get Me Back is an online community for women getting fit after cancer, run by cancer fitness specialist Sarah Newman: getmeback.uk

Headwrappers is a hair loss advisory service, focusing on alternatives to wigs such as headscarves: headwrappers.org

Life After Cancer runs courses and support groups supporting adults to increase their mental wellbeing after cancer: life-aftercancer.co.uk

LoveRose is luxury lingerie cleverly designed for post-breast surgery: loveroselingerie.com

Macmillan helpline for practical advice on things like financial support during treatment: 0808 808 0000, macmillan.org.uk

Maggie's helpline to find out about your nearest centre and what they offer: 0300 123 1801, maggies.org

Menopause and Cancer Chat Hub on Facebook, for Dani Binnington's post-cancer menopause support community

Paxman's guide to Scalp Cooling Technology: coldcap.com

Penny Brohn UK helps people live well with cancer, through online group sessions and workshops at their centre in Bristol: pennybrohn.org.uk

Seasonal eating: guide to seasonal eating at vegsoc.org or eattheseasons.co.uk

SMILES trial, proving the link between good nutrition and mental health. More information can be found at foodandmoodcentre.com.au/smiles-trial

Trekstock is a great charity for people under 40 with cancer: trekstock.com

Wellness for Cancer is a US-based charity that provides training to beauty and massage therapists globally: w4cancer.com

Yes to Life is an integrative care charity, providing support to cancer patients seeking to pursue approaches currently only available privately: 0870 163 2990, yestolife.org.uk

Acknowledgements

Without Katya Shipster, my editor at HarperCollins, this book wouldn't exist. Thank you for being so honest and generous with your time, your ideas and your own experience. And for being such a powerful model of living well beyond breast cancer, with your joyous energy (and the best nails in publishing).

Thank you to the dream team at HarperCollins: Isabel Prodger, Hattie Evans, Sarah Hammond.

To Viola Hayden, my radiant and inspiring agent.

To *Sunday Times Style* editor Laura Atkinson, who commissioned the column that sparked hundreds of messages from readers, clearly showing why this book is so necessary.

To all the women from whom I learnt to put myself back together, who I met through support groups, workshops and on Instagram. There are too many to mention, but special thanks to Carly Moosah, Emma McCarthy, Helen Addis, Leah Hardy, Sarah Newman, Liz O'Riordan, Toral Shah, Natalie Hall and Dani Binnington.

Most of all, thank you to Jonathan, Ezra and Eden, for everything.

About the Author

Rosamund Dean is a journalist, author and former deputy editor of *Grazia*. In 2021, she was diagnosed with breast cancer at the age of 40 and documented her journey with a column in the *Sunday Times Style*. She has since founded Well Well Well, a popular wellness newsletter on Substack, chronicling her efforts to future-proof her body in a way that is relatable and doable. She is also the author of *Mindful Drinking: How Cutting Down Can Change Your Life*.

Rosamund lives in London with her husband, *Sunday Times* writer Jonathan Dean, and their two children.